THE AGE OF
GLOBESITY

Entering the Perfect Storm

The Complete Resource for the Low Glycemic Index

PATINO DIET

FRANK PATINO, M.D.
& HENRY PATINO

The advice offered in this book, although based on the author's personal and clinical experience, is not intended to be a substitute for the advice and counsel of a personal physician. If you are currently taking diuretics, insulin, or oral diabetes medications, consult your physician before starting the PATINO DIET. You will need to reduce and then closely monitor your dosage as you lower your blood sugar level. People with severe kidney disease should not attempt the PATINO DIET. The weight loss phases of the PATINO DIET are not appropriate for pregnant women or nursing mothers.

THE AGE OF GLOBESITY: ENTERING THE PERFECT STORM – **THE COMPLETE RESOURCE FOR THE LOW GLYCEMIC INDEX PATINO DIET.**

For more information:
ATTN: Globesity LLC
29150 Buckingham St., Suite # 6
Livonia MI 48154

Library of Congress Cataloging-in-Publication Data

Patino, Frank
   The Age of Globesity
   p. tp.
   Original Publication: Michigan, 2013
   Includes biographical references and index.
   ISBN #
   1. Reducing diets. 2. Low-carbohydrate diet 3. Low glycemic diet. I. Title: The Age of Globesity. II. Title: Entering the Perfect Storm. III. Title: The Complete Resource for the Low Glycemic Index Patino Diet

LOC Codes
###

Acknowledgements

This work would not have come into being without the assistance and guidance of my family.

Krystal I hope this book
will set a foundation
for a healthier future.
God Bless,
Paul

Table of Contents

INSPIRATION

RISKS

HOW IT WORKS

THE SCIENCE

THE PATINO DIET

Introduction

Our world is entering a new age - the Age of Globesity. Like a perfect storm, obesity and the inevitable medical repercussions accompanying it are bringing our economies to the breaking point. Most of us are blissfully unaware of the danger that lies ahead.

For thirty years now the medical profession has become more and more alarmed at the rise in cardiovascular disease and the lethal toll it has taken on our culture. Attempts to curb this ominous cloud growing in the horizon have met with little success.

Every year the number of diabetics continues to escalate. At one time type II diabetes was known as adult onset

The irony is that we now have more than ever, and yet this may end up killing us.

diabetes. The disease typically emerged in adults that had become obese and after some time, fell victim to the horrendous liabilities of type 2 diabetes. We are finding that as obesity begins to increase in children, type 2 diabetes can no longer be called adult onset.

An alarming rise in diseases, which are ironically related to lifestyle excesses, is beginning to take an increasing toll on the health and vitality of our nation. The steady rise in the incidences of cardiovascular disease, diabetes, myocardial infarctions, strokes, cancer and perhaps even Alzheimer's, which we are experiencing in the western nations, can be directly or indirectly related to obesity. Unfortunately, these are generally caused by incorrect diets, over-consumption, and exercise deprivation.

The medical ramifications of starting down this slippery slope at younger ages are horrendous, not only to the individual but to the cost of medical treatment and for society as a whole. Medical insurance will soar through the roof in order to pay for this approaching, perfect storm.

Sadly, most who are attempting to overcome this problem are in fact adding to it through the use of high glycemic carbohydrate diets, which they erroneously think will help them lose weight.

Little is understood of the role that insulin plays in this unfolding drama. Little is understood about the importance of the glycemic index in this regard. This book will help the reader understand the secret of losing the midriff fat that leads to these serious health problems.

Sadly, the vast majority of people that are obese have tried countless fad diets in desperate attempts to lose weight. Most have failed, not because they did not try, but because the diets were unwittingly helping them to store more fat rather than burning it as fuel.

Their will to overcome obstacles has been dealt a severe blow by the constant failures of the past. But there is hope. This book has been written to give you that hope. We know a little about overcoming obstacles and hope that our story can inspire you and educate you to become victorious.

We have found that adversity is what brings forth character and character is what breeds success.

Inspiration

Overcoming

There are obstacles in our lives that may seem insurmountable to us. Like torpedoes that appear an instant before the explosion, our lives can be hit broadside. In a single heartbeat our long accustomed routine may be changed forever. What will we do when such drastic events knock us off our feet?

I heard my little brother Billy describe his profession once, "Being a pilot is 99% sheer boredom, and 1% sheer panic." I think that for most of us, this describes our lives. Most of us go about our daily mundane routines almost in automatic pilot mode. But here and there, certain obstacles come into our lives that can cause us to crash and burn, which demand our immediate and undivided attention if we hope to stay the course. Unfortunately, obstacles are a very real part of each and every one of our lives. No one is exempt.

Some obstacles are like icebergs, almost completely submerged with only a small visible sign above the surface of the impending doom below it. If we are careful to maintain a vigil, we can spot them in the distance and veer safely around them. Others, however, like a torpedo to our broadside, are wholly unavoidable and leave us no recourse but to persevere through them. My grandfather used to say, "It's not the obstacles in one's life that defines a person, but how he overcomes them."

Life can come at us quick, and in a single heartbeat our lives can be completely changed forever. Those of us who watched the downing of the Twin Towers in quiet desperation and unbelief can appreciate this reality. Who would have thought that the destruction of two buildings could have affected our culture so deeply? We will never be the same. These torpedoes to our broadside, if they do not kill us, may sometimes be an opportunity for us to make lemonade out of lemons.

My early childhood experiences were filled with happiness. I lived in a paradise, which I naively believed would last forever. Our family owned a large sugar cane plantation in Cuba.   We were well-to-do and lived quite comfortably. The freedom I enjoyed romping on the farm with my brothers and cousins gave me the impression that I lived in paradise.

My first encounter with one of life's unavoidable obstacles came when I was just six years old. That fateful day on April 19, 1961, I saw a military Jeep, with an army truck following close behind it, pull up in front of my house. A dozen militiamen scrambled out the back of the truck with rifles and machine guns at the ready and proceeded to surround our house.

The lieutenant in the Jeep pulled out his revolver from his holster, walked to our front door, and knocked loudly using the handle butt of his gun. "Paco, we wish to speak to you!" A friend in the police headquarters had previously warned my father that they were coming to arrest him and had advised him to run. But my father chose not to flee. He refused to leave his six children and his American wife at the mercy of Castro's men.

A few minutes before the militiamen arrived, my father had warned my mother of the events that would shortly unfold. She was now crying uncontrollably by his side as they handcuffed him and took him away. I did not quite understand what was going on at that time, but I knew instinctively that my paradise had ended.

My father had been a gunrunner for the underground resistance against Castro's communist dictatorship before the ill-fated Bay of Pigs Invasion. One of the members of his underground group had been arrested and had ratted out the rest of the group. Dad had been singled out as one of the leaders.

I watched in horror as the militiamen ransacked our house looking for evidence, until they finally drove off with Dad in the backseat of the Jeep. As the dust of the tires from the speeding Jeep kicked up in a cloud, Dad turned his head and looked back at us, for one last glance, before disappearing around the corner. I did not know what fate awaited him, but I later found out what had happened to him on that fateful day.

Dad was taken to the edge of one of the sugar cane fields. The men scrambled out of the truck again and promptly assembled into a firing squad formation. Dad was roughly removed from the Jeep and placed in front of them, with a blindfold. The lieutenant shouted with authority, "Ready... aim........" and paused for effect. Then he said, "Paco, I will give you one chance to save your life. I need you to name all the men who were in your group." But my father put on his best poker face, insisting that he was being framed because they wanted to take over his farm.

The officer said, "Fine, then we will continue with the execution. Ready...aim............fire!" The guns roared, and the bullets whizzed by, over the top of my father's head. "I will give you one last chance, Paco," said the young officer. "If you refuse to cooperate, you will force me to do what I do not wish to do."

"I am being framed, I tell you. I have no idea what you are talking about." Dad knew that if he talked, others would die as well.

"Very well." The anger and frustration in the officer's voice was now clearly evident. "Men, get ready... aim.......... fire!"

But the bullets whizzed by above his head again. Still my father continued with his charade. The frustrated young lieutenant finally realized that Dad was not going to spill the beans. Yanking the blindfold off his head, he pushed him back in the Jeep and drove him to prison.

My father was 35 years old with jet-black hair when they arrested him, in the prime of his life. Three months later, he was still being detained in San Severin Prison located in the Cuban Province of Matanzas. The prisoners were poorly fed, and for this reason they allowed their families to visit occasionally to bring some much-needed food, medicines and vitamins.

Each prisoner was allowed one java, which is a paper bag with rope handles attached to it. Since only a few visitors were allowed per prisoner, my mother decided it was best to take my oldest brother Henry with her.

San Severin was an old Spanish dungeon that had been converted into a prison. A ramp extending around the top of the wall was filled with visitors anxiously waiting to see their loved ones. The open court below was filled with the prisoners milling about in their khaki colored uniforms.

Henry peered over the wall to the crowd of prisoners below, scanning for my father. "Where is he? I can't find him!"

My mother leaned down and pointed, "There he is!"

But Henry was still unable to recognize him.

"There he is!" Then she paused briefly, realizing why Henry could not recognize him. "His hair is white now, but don't tell him that we noticed it." My dad's hair had turned completely white in a few months' time.

In a single instant, our lives had changed forever. We had taken a torpedo broadside and our ship was in danger of sinking. How does a wife take care of six children while her husband is in political prison? She is now an enemy of the state and cannot work. How can she survive?

After the Bay of Pigs Invasion, which took place not more than twenty kilometers from a section of our farm, my mom thought it best to move my family to Havana to be with her parents.

Abuelo (grandfather) and Abuela (grandmother) lived directly in front of the American Embassy, overlooking the ocean. On my tiptoes, I could see over their fourth floor balcony as the waves crashed unto the malecon (the sea wall), spraying foam skyward ten to fifteen feet, and spilling into the street. "Where is America, Abuelo?"

Abuelo would point to the ocean's northern horizon and say, "It is that way, but it is so far that you cannot see it from here."

My world had changed drastically. The days of roaming freely through the farm were now replaced by living in a crowded city apartment with only two bedrooms. Instead of freedom and joy, my heart was filled with anguish and the uncertainty of not knowing if I would ever see my father or my family's farm again.

Dad had made my grandfather promise him that if anything were to happen to him, he would take Mom and the children to the United States, where they would be safe. My mother at first resisted. She felt that she would be abandoning Dad if she left for America. But when the American Embassy was ousted from Cuba, she finally relented and decided for our sakes to do as my father wished. We would have to leave all that my family had worked for behind.

Sadness was etched in my mother's face as we drove silently to the airport that day. I had never been on an airplane before, and I had no idea how long this flight was going to take to reach that mythical faraway land called America. I only knew that America was so far away that I could not even see her from the height of Abuelo's apartment. I asked my mother, "Mom how many days will we be flying?"

She laughed, and for a few precious moments her anguish gave way to her beautiful smile. "God willing, we will be there by tonight," she answered.

We had brought our suitcases with clothes and many of our family photographs, along with a few items of personal value, but we were not allowed to keep anything. They took everything we had at the airport, even my mother's wedding ring, which made her cry. All we were left with was the clothes we wore on our backs. Abuelo said that it did not matter, because we were flying to freedom. On June 30, 1961, my family arrived in Miami, Florida, while my father remained imprisoned in Cuba.

How quickly life comes at you, and in a single heartbeat our lives can change forever. Some obstacles we have power to avoid and change. Others, like a torpedo to our broadside, we cannot avoid. In these difficult and painful times, we must persevere and endure, if we hope to come out on the other side. This life-lesson we learned as we left behind all that we owned and held dear to come to the land of freedom. But how do you prepare for the unexpected? How do you endure a path that will bring great suffering in unfamiliar territory?

Our family learned that together we could overcome any obstacles that came our way. We learned the power of accountability to one another. We learned that together we could conquer the seemingly insurmountable.

My first night in America was frightening. Having been inoculated while going through U.S. Customs, some of us were running fevers. My Aunt Tati and my paternal grandmother, Mema, had moved to Miami two years prior, after my paternal grandfather, Pepe, had passed away with cancer. They had rented an apartment on South West 8th Street, now notoriously famous as the Cuban district called *Calle Ocho*. Across from them, on the north side of the street, was a Pizza Palace, with waitresses on skates and dressed in shorts, bringing trays that hook to the car doors. The jukebox in this popular restaurant played loud pop music incessantly until the wee-hours of the morning.

We were too many to fit in the modest two-bedroom apartment of my Aunt Tati, so my grandfather rented a room in a nearby cheap motel called El Nido, "the nest." At that age, I had no clue what the name insinuated. I thought the owner must love birds. Many years later, I visited the small motel and rented the room for the night, in remembrance of that day. It seemed so much smaller than I had remembered.

The sweltering heat and suffocating humidity so typical of the Miami I grew to love seemed to me to be particularly brutal that first night. Aunt Tati's apartment had no air conditioning. My older brothers, Henry and Robert, and my sister, Nena, slept in my aunt's apartment with the windows open to the roaring traffic outside. However, I was fortunate enough to sleep in the very small efficiency motel room with Abuelo and Abuela, which at least had air conditioning. Mike, Joe and I slept on cushions on the floor.

Henry later confessed to me that he was not able to sleep a single wink that night. The loud BOOM BOOM of the jukebox, the sound of the whisking cars, the horns, the headlights flashing across the walls of the room, the sirens in the background were all so unfamiliar to those of us who were raised on the farm. In the little paradise we had left behind, all one could hear in the night was an occasional rooster in the distance or the distant bark of a dog. But most of the time, all one could hear was the musical sound of crickets, which fills the night air with their soothing background melody. If it had rained during the day, then the croaking song of the frogs would sound in synchrony with the crickets, creating an enchanting symphony that seemed to magically soothe my soul. Even our sky seemed to contain more stars. I later learned that the city lights mask all but the brightest stars.

Abuelo managed to find an old, three bedroom, wooden house that we could rent, only a few blocks from my aunt's apartment. Abuelo and Abuela slept in one room. My mom and sister Isabel (Nena) were in another, smaller room. And all four of my brothers and I slept in the third room. I don't know why, but all of us had nicknames while growing up in Cuba, which we quickly discarded in America. Henry (Kike) and Mike (Mini) slept in the same bed. Robert (Teto) and Joe (Pepi) slept in another. And I (Pancho) slept in an aluminum foldout cot, wedged between the two beds.

Each night before going to bed, my mother gathered us together, and we prayed for God to watch over Dad and bring him back to us safely. Immediately afterwards, I would take a cold shower and rush to go to sleep before the heat would cause me to break out into an uncomfortable sweat, which would keep me awake.

Two months later, it was time to start the school year. Just four short months prior, I had been roaming carefree in my little paradise. Now, we were being taken to Auburndale Elementary School for our first day in an American school. Although my grandparents and my mom spoke English fluently, none of us knew how to speak a single word of English. It was convenient for the adults in Cuba to break into English when they did not want the children to know what they were talking about.

We had arrived in America in one of the first waves of Cuban immigrants that swarmed into Miami during those years. When my mom dropped me off in Mrs. Madison's classroom, I was the only Cuban student and my 30 classmates spoke only English. That first day at school I cried from the moment my mom left me to the moment I saw her again. Mrs. Madison was certainly a very nice teacher, and she tried her best to console me. She would come and speak softly to me, but I had not a single clue what she was saying and that only made me cry even more. The children would attempt to talk to me, but I could not respond. I just simply cried.

But I was not alone. My older brother Henry later confessed to me that he was equally terrified. That day, he was taken to the school cafeteria along with approximately 150 other students who also only spoke English. The teacher spoke through a microphone as the students sat, six to a table. Henry was sitting in the very back, next to the exit door. As the morning wore on, he needed to go to the bathroom but he did not know how to ask the teacher to be excused. Squirming nervously in his seat, he held it for as long as he could until he simply wet his pants. Mortified, burying his head in his arms, he thought, "If the other students see me, I will always be known as the kid that wet his pants!"

When they took a few minutes of recess, Henry would not get up from his chair and risk that anyone would see that his pants were wet. Fortunately, that first day of orientation only lasted until noon. When at long last the dismissal bell went off, he tore out of the school running like a bat out of hell and did not stop until he reached our house. That day, Abuelo taught him how to say, "May I please be excused?"

After a few months, a few more Cubans had arrived and joined my burgeoning class, at which time they assigned Miss Garcia, as Mrs. Madison's assistant, to be our teacher. Within a year, I was speaking fluent English and was able to return to the regular classroom.

Life had changed dramatically for us in a few short months and things would never be the same. We were used to roaming carefree on the farm, with maids and nannies to look after us. Now, we lived in a strange country where we did not speak the language and we were dirt poor.

My mother needed to find a job to support us. She bought an old portable Smith Corona manual typewriter, the kind that you had to push the keys all the way down to print. She bought a few books and taught herself to type and write in shorthand. Soon after, she landed a job with the U.S. government as a clerk. She retired a few years ago, after working for 35 years as a GS-13. She was the personal secretary to the South East Regional head of the Equal Employment Opportunity Commission.

All of us had to pitch in and help with the house chores. Nena would often cook for us while mom worked. Money was tight in those days, and there was precious little available for buying the clothes that were popular with our fellow students. We mostly wore hand-me-downs. Some students in school would make fun of our raggedy clothes, so we decided that we would earn the money to buy our own clothes.

It was during that time, in the early Sixties, that gasoline-powered lawn mowers were becoming popular in Miami. Robert found an old cylindrical push-mower, which had been discarded in the trash, and brought it home. Robert and Henry took it apart, cleaned all the rust from it, greased the gears, and sharpened the blades. Abuelo bought us a brand new rake, and we set off through the neighborhood knocking on every door. "Mam wan gras cut, fisty sens."

Robert and Henry would take turns pushing the mower, and I would rake after them. Eventually, we were able to buy one of those "Red Flyer" wagons, which we brought with us in order to collect any fruits from the yards that we cut. In this way, we were able to sell a variety of fruits to other neighbors and increase our profit. Grapefruits, oranges, mangoes, and avocadoes were ten cents. Lemons and limes were only a nickel apiece.

We collected soda pop bottles from the playground and newspapers that had been thrown in the trash. Using wood from crates that had been discarded by a glass company, and metal sheets that had been discarded by a printing shop, we constructed a little storage area behind our home where we could store the papers and keep them dry. When a significant amount had been collected, Abuela would drive us to the recycling center, where we would get paid for the material we brought in.

With this money we were able to purchase some of the clothes we wanted, plus a brand new, green bike with a white cushioned banana seat and high handlebars. Unfortunately, our very first bike was later stolen. From then on we bought locks and chains. In spite of this disappointment, we learned some valuable lessons. Abuelo taught us that in this great country, if you are willing to work hard enough, with perseverance, tenacity, and determination, anyone could achieve whatever goals he sets for himself.

But I have also grown to understand that some things are beyond our scope to accomplish in our own power. There was nothing that we could do to bring our father back. Mom taught us that in these things, we had to trust God. Each night, without fail, our family gathered before bedtime and prayed.

In April of 1966, Dad was eventually released from prison after serving a five-year sentence and enduring many hardships. Our first prayer was answered; he made it out of prison alive. Our second prayer was for God to bring him to us in America. We expected this to be a long and arduous procedure, with little realistic chance of it coming to pass. But God's grace smiled down upon our family. It was precisely during this time that the Freedom Flights had been arranged between America and Cuba.

Just three months after being set free from prison, in July of 1966, Dad was able to come to the United States. I remember waiting by a chain link fence for him to be released, after going through security debriefing at the airport. When he came through the gate, I hardly remembered what his face looked like. Mike and Joe did not remember him at all. They were too young when he was taken from us. Our second prayer was answered. We were poor, but we were together. One more obstacle was conquered.

We had lost everything we owned, our paradise, our family wealth, our home, and even our family films and photographs from our childhood, but we had each other. For Dad, the challenges that lay before him were no less than the rigors he had to endure in the past. Now, my father needed to find employment.

Soon after he arrived, he was asked to go to Nicaragua, in order to manage sugar cane farms owned by General Somoza. It was a tempting offer that would have provided handsomely for him, but Dad was not fond of dictators, even if they had helped the exiled community during the Bay of Pigs Invasion. He chose instead to work in a kitchen cabinet factory, sweeping floors in order to give his children the benefit of the freedoms afforded by this great nation. His selfless sacrifice was an important life lesson that penetrated deep into all of us. We adjusted to the American culture and all of us became American citizens by choice, not through happenstance of birth.

After graduating from Miami Senior High School, I was accepted to the University of Miami pre-med program. My family had no money to help me with my tuition. I was hired by the Miami Beach Fire Department, where I became a firefighter/paramedic. This allowed me to work my way through school. I have always wanted to work in a profession that would help people, and working as a firefighter and paramedic allowed me to do just that. It also gave me an understanding of the medical field from a unique perspective, as a first responder.

I went to school part-time, often trading shifts with other firefighters in order to get the days I needed to attend my classes. I was also fortunate to have an understanding fire chief, who allowed me to serve as a physical training instructor for the new recruits. Instead of paying me for my time, I was given time off to go to school. It was an arduous and seemingly endless route. After finally graduating from the University of Miami, I was accepted to the University of Florida College of Medicine. I reluctantly retired from the Fire Department, which I had grown to love, and used the money I had saved in my pension, plus a number of student loans, to pay for my tuition.

By this time, I had married and my son Franky had been born. It is hard enough to go through school as a single person, but to attempt it while you still have to provide for a family is ridiculous. Those were lean days financially, and my family would, as often as they could, send me money to survive. I have learned throughout the years that the most important thing in life is my family.

We are not a perfect family. There are no perfect families. But our family has learned to band together against the storms of life. We have reached out to help each other in times of need. We have learned to overcome together. We learned during this experience that the conquest of those seemingly insurmountable obstacles could best be executed if we turn to our family as a unit and become personally accountable.

Most people facing problems of obesity, drug dependency, or any other seemingly insurmountable medical situation, do not establish a system of personal accountability. They, like all the rest of us, are predisposed to avoid accountability. We have become hyper-individualists with thick walls around us to guard from any authority structures or potential interference with our unrestrained ego.

The day of my graduation my family drove up from Miami to Gainesville, Florida for the ceremony. Afterwards, my mother was crying as she pulled me to her and kissed me. But then she surprised me completely when she began to apologize profusely. With tears in her eyes and an occasional sob, she said, "I am so sorry that we failed you guys as parents to provide the financial support for your education. I feel so guilty!" I was dumbstruck. Dad also has had great difficulty dealing with the guilt that our family fortune was lost during his watch. But these are the torpedoes to our broadside that we have no power to avoid.

"Mom," I said, "what are you talking about? What you gave us is more valuable than all the money in the world! You and Dad taught us to never give up, no matter how hard things got, no matter how dark things turned. No matter how many times we fall, you taught us to simply stand up again, dust ourselves off, and keep on plugging. You taught us that if we worked hard enough we could accomplish whatever goals we set for ourselves. You gave us hope in the midst of darkness. You taught us to be accountable to one another and that is what made us overcome our own personal obstacles. Dad taught us, not just with words, but also with his life, to stand against evil, no matter the cost. To fight for your family and your nation's freedom, even against insurmountable odds. You both showed us the meaning of love by the way you sacrificed for us. You taught us by your example the meaning of a family. You gave us exactly what we needed to survive in this world. You are no failure, you are the best parents that anyone could ever want, and my brothers and I, are, of all people, the most fortunate in the world to have had you as our parents!"

Later on, I pondered what I might have become if things had been different. When on that fateful day, in April of 1961, my paradise was lost and my dad was taken from my family, we received a torpedo broadside that we had no power to avoid. But we persevered, and what was meant for evil, God had turned for good.

Some obstacles we can avoid, but those we cannot we must endure in hope and never give up. We must establish a group around us that we can be accountable to and day-by-day deal with the problem. In the blink of an eye, all of our worldly goods can be taken from us, but our possessions do not define us. We may learn that we have cancer. We may have a heart attack. We may learn that we are now diabetics. How do we overcome such torpedoes in our lives?

I have learned that the obstacles are not what define us. The choices that we make are what define us. This was my first epiphany.

Our Human Family

My second epiphany came to me in the face of a little boy. After I finished my residency and fellowship, in order to pay off my tuition loans, I would fly as often as possible with a local air ambulance company to earn extra pay. Most of the flights were to the Caribbean and Central and South America to pick up either Canadian or American tourists and bring them to the States or back to Canada for medical treatment. I flew about 200 missions total during that time, which gave me a real understanding of the impoverished living conditions that exist outside of our great nation.

Most of us in America have no idea of the tremendous difficulties that many human beings suffer outside of our country. We scarcely appreciate the freedoms our nation provides and take for granted the relative prosperity created by those freedoms.

We were flying in a Leer jet to Honduras one particular day to pick up an American that had become gravely ill. As we made the final approach to the airport, I looked out of the window and saw small, scattered fires that spotted the landscape with plumes of smoke as far as the eye could see. Military trucks and personnel were milling everywhere through hundreds of these billowing columns of smoke. The men were armed to the teeth, and the area literally looked like the battle zones I had only seen in movies. I leaned into the cockpit and asked the pilots, "What in the world is going on down there?" They had no clue either, but the airport authorities assured us that it was safe to land.

After we landed, an armed officer came to the airplane and brought a full military escort with him to take us to the hospital. They were instructed to escort us under armed guards so that we could pick up our patient safely. The guards immediately set up a military perimeter around us, while the officer explained the situation.

It seems that the communists had been fomenting violence in the Mayan Indian community by spreading false propaganda. They were claiming that Americans were kidnapping their children in order to use their organs for spare parts in America. In turn, the Mayans were kidnapping and killing Americans in revenge.

As the officer was speaking, I caught the eye of a barefoot, dirty-faced little boy who must have been about five years old, the same age as my son Franky at the time. I remember thinking how his face looked like Linus in the Snoopy cartoons, except that his eyes were filled with anguish and suffering. The little boy stared blankly at me with a forlorn look on his face.

I became totally transfixed on that fragile and undernourished little boy. All of the sounds around me faded as I looked into his dark, languid eyes. The boy walked slowly toward me, with his right arm outstretched and palm cupped upward. He walked right through the perimeter of the soldiers without them even noticing, almost as if he were invisible. He stepped in front of me with his outstretched arm and simply looked into my eyes, without saying a single word.

I leaned down to his level, held his hand and smiled at him. Then I took out my wallet, gave him some money, and told him in Spanish to go buy some food. The old seasoned nurse that had flown there with me said gruffly, "What a softy, you shouldn't encourage these beggars. You will only teach them to beg more."

I turned in anger to her, trying to contain myself, and said, "It is one thing to beg in a place where there is work and opportunity to better oneself. It is completely another to live in a place where there is no opportunity to climb from the squalor of poverty. This poor boy is obviously undernourished and suffering greatly. I lost nothing by freely giving him what God has freely given me. He could have been my own son, if I had but been born here."

That night, when I finally arrived home at about 3:30 in the morning, I went to my son's bedroom and knelt next to his bed as he peacefully slept, unaware of the tumult in my heart. I kissed him gently so as not to not wake him, and I thanked my God that my son had a warm bed, a roof over his head, and that he never had to go hungry. As I slipped into bed, my wife woke up and I shared my story with her. I felt that I was the luckiest man on earth.

The eyes and face of that little boy have forever been engrained in my mind. I knew right then and there that I had to be involved in something that would attempt to reach out to the children in need, in these Third World nations wallowing in such abject poverty. But what?

Not long after, my dad called me on the phone and explained to me that he felt he needed to do something to help the families of political prisoners in Cuba. The living conditions for most Cubans had deteriorated greatly since the lethal talons of communism gripped the island, and many were in great need of the basic necessities of life. But the family members of political prisoners are in the worst situation possible in the whole of the communist island. They are no longer entitled to medical care from the government, and employment is next to impossible for them.

They are the disenfranchised and forgotten members of our extended human family, caught in a relentless limbo. Their principle breadwinner has been locked up for political reasons and is therefore incapable of caring for them. "We must do something," said Dad. He wanted to begin sending them medicines. I was working for Pfizer Corporation at the time, and so I approached the company about donating medicines.

My dad, my brothers, and I incorporated a non-profit organization named Health Help Project, and we began to send medicines to Cuba. We wanted our organization to be run and operated with 100% volunteer workers and no paid staff. All of us had been so disgusted by some of the organizations whose staff members made extravagant salaries, eating up much of the donated proceeds that ought to have been given to the needy. We wanted every penny that was donated to our organization to be sent to the poor.

Soon, we were getting donations of all kinds of medical equipment and supplies from hospitals all over the place. Most of these were things that we could not send to Cuba, because the government officials would confiscate them for their own use. So we began to establish contacts with other non-profit organizations inside poverty-stricken countries, in order to bypass their local politicians, who, for the most part, historically, would rob most of the stuff and sell it in the black market.

We had no fancy advertising campaigns and no Madison Avenue promoters. Word spread from one volunteer to another, and before we knew it we were sending millions of dollars of medical supplies and equipment to clinics every year and outfitting hospitals and clinics in the rural areas of these poverty stricken nations. Soon we were sending equipment to 17 different countries and even bringing in children to have operations performed here in America. It is truly amazing to see how God has engineered all of this on a shoestring budget, and the labor of love of many wonderful volunteers.

Our family is grateful to God for the many blessings He has given us, and we simply wanted to give back to those who were less fortunate, a little of what He has freely given to us. This is my second epiphany. I have come to understand that these disenfranchised members of our human family are the people facing obstacles, which they cannot veer from. They have received a torpedo to the broadside, and there are no lifeboats left for them. They are swimming in the deep dark waters of life without hope that anything will ever be different.

We can provide for them vital help to safely navigate the lethal waters to safe harbor with only a little sacrifice, effort, and time to help them persevere; to help them become self-reliant. Sadly, most of us living in comfort do not want to be bothered by the suffering of others. We are reticent to engage ourselves in anything that would require any sacrifice of us. It has been my experience that those who have never really experienced suffering rarely care about those who do. But if we care enough to take the scale from our eyes and learn to be a little selfless, we can change the future for others, one life at a time.

What works for our immediate family also works for our extended family. Modern science has empirically evidenced the fact that a single matriarch engendered all of humanity. Whether the reader believes that an Almighty Creator created mankind, or that mankind is the product of the evolutionary process, the fact remains we are all descended from a single ancestral mother.

Studies of mitochondrial DNA have conclusively shown that the differences between us are so minute as to be practically negligible. If this is true, then we are truly one family. We are all brothers and sisters who are trapped in this spinning rock and struggling to survive. How, then, can we not help one another? Strangers are after all only family members that we have yet to meet and know.

I have learned that our human tendency to be selfish is the cause of the many injustices that exploit the disenfranchised members of our global human family. Selfishness is the culprit that brings about great suffering and pain. It is the engine of injustice that allows the powerful to prey upon the weak. But what could I do to change the world?

I realized that I could not change the world, but I could change myself. I could learn to become a little less selfish every day. I could learn to sacrifice for others a little bit at a time. I could help others to watch out for the icebergs and help them, as best I could when they were torpedoed. This was my second epiphany.

The Curse of Plenty

There are some, who have learned the indispensable necessity of being vigilant in order to see that iceberg, warning us of the looming danger hiding below the surface. Wise is the person who can foresee danger and steer clear of it for his family's safety. But we must be willing and capable of recognizing the signs of danger in order to safely veer from the path that may bring disaster.

Since that second epiphany, I have grown to understand that those who do without are not the only ones faced with great danger. Our nation, which abounds in plenty, is also heading into a "perfect storm," not because of lack but ironically because of plenty.

Sadly, most Americans are woefully unaware of monstrous icebergs lurking in their paths, dangers that I foresee will bring tragedy to many families. I am deeply concerned for the welfare of my nation. Our affluence has brought with it attendant dangers equally as destructive and equally as lethal as those which accompany hunger and poverty.

Our concern for the poor should not waiver, but it is becoming apparent that we need to be concerned for the wealthy as well. The gap between the rich and poor grows wider with each passing year. This social and economic gap between the world's richest 1 billion people and the world's poorest 1 billion people has no historical precedent in recorded human history.

At the bottom end of the spectrum, the disenfranchised members of our human family struggle for daily survival. The lack of daily sustenance at the most basic level, food and clean water, leaves them precariously vulnerable to opportunistic diseases. The U.N. Food and Agriculture Organization has reported that there are 862 million members of our human family who are presently undernourished and chronically hungry. The children are the innocent victims who are most acutely impacted by this tragedy. Malnutrition stunts their growth, curtails their mental capacity, and compromises their immune systems. As a direct consequence, they are more severely plagued and overcome by such infectious diseases as malaria, tuberculosis, dysentery, measles, respiratory infections, and AIDS, which typically torment the poor disproportionately to the rest of society.

The lack of clean water, which we take for granted in the western world, is a major global health problem. Waterborne diseases such as cholera, dysentery, and a host of parasites claim more than 3 million precious lives each passing year. For this reason, the average life expectancy in the poorest nations is only around 40 years.

In the west, modern advancements in medicine and farming techniques have resulted in an average life expectancy that now incredibly ranges around 80 years of age. The use of irrigation pumps and the mechanization of farming tools, as well as the use of fertilizers and pesticides due to the availability of cheap oil in the twentieth century, have provided unprecedented agricultural yields in the majority of the western world. The skyrocketing cost of fossil fuel will most certainly impact this present bounty in the future, but for now our land is certainly a veritable horn of plenty.

However, for this segment of our human family that has reaped the benefits of this technology, new evidence indicates that an ominous rise in disease will shortly begin to reverse the trend toward increased longevity. There is a hidden danger that may threaten, and even reverse, the magnificent advancements made through our modern technology.

In addition to the already well-documented health problems resulting from the ingestion of carcinogens, such as those found in tobacco products, air pollution, and foods laced with pesticides, there is an iceberg of unprecedented proportions that is looming ever larger in the near horizon. The iceberg is obesity.

An alarming rise in diseases related to lifestyle excesses is beginning to take an increasing toll on the health and vitality of our nation. The steady rise in the incidence of cardiovascular disease, diabetes, myocardial infarctions, strokes, and perhaps even Alzheimer's, which we are experiencing in the western nations, can be directly or indirectly related to obesity, which in turn is generally caused by incorrect diets, over-consumption, and exercise deprivation.

Most Americans are blindly navigating in due course to crash and sink, completely unaware of the lethal consequences they will face in the future because of their poor choices today. These choices are not being made out of selfishness, but out of ignorance. For this reason I have chosen to write this book in order to sound the alarm, in the hopes that some will open their eyes and change their course before it is too late.

The social and economic impact of this escalating trend in obesity is not being greatly appreciated by most in our western culture. It will probably continue to be ignored by most of us until the lethal consequences strikes one in our family. In a single heartbeat our lives can change forever, but it need not be gloom and doom. It can change for good, or it can change for bad.

Our choices have consequences. If we learn to make the right choices, we can hedge our bets against many of the billowing storms of life. We can avoid many of those hidden obstacles that lead to suffering and pain, if we recognize the dangers early enough to make the right corrections to our path.

The collective fate of our nation rests on the individual choices that we will make in the near future. The right choices will lead to healthy and productive lives, which naturally results in a prosperous nation. The wrong choices will bring upon us illness, disability, and even death before our time. Sadly, it shall be the ruin of many families. Moreover, it shall certainly result in the financial ruin of our entire nation, if we do not recognize the problem at hand and properly address it before it is too late. The choice is ours to make.

For the past several decades America has been making a series of bad choices in several separate and yet related areas that are driving us toward that iceberg. This perfect storm has the potential of financially sinking our nation, and ruining the lives of many individuals and families. It is this realization that brought me to my third epiphany.

The Coming Perfect Storm

My third epiphany came to me in a water park in Detroit, Michigan. It was nearing the end of a long cold winter in Michigan, and it had been too many days since I had spent quality time with my ten-year-old daughter. I was looking forward to taking a break from my highly stressful life and turning the gears off in my brain, which had for too long been smoking in overdrive.

Raised in Miami, I have missed the relaxing benefit of its famous sun, sand, and surf, which I no longer take for granted. So Sarah and I decided to go to an indoor water park for some long overdue rest and relaxation. It wouldn't be Miami, but it was better than shoveling snow.

Sarah and I eagerly anticipated using the two large water slides at the enormous facility. As we walked into the massive indoor swimming area, I smelled the humid, chlorine-tainted odor so familiar to me. It brought a flood of memories from my childhood at Shenandoah Pool, where I learned to swim. But as I looked up, I was stopped dead in my tracks by the almost surreal scene that loomed before me.

In my early 20's, while working my way through college and before becoming a firefighter, I had worked as a lifeguard captain at John U. Lloyd State Park in Florida. Needless to say, I am no stranger to crowded bathing areas. However, I was not prepared for the shock that awaited me at this water park.

The area was teeming with hundreds of screaming children and adults romping in the water, but it wasn't the size of the crowd or the intensity of the noise that shocked me. As I surveyed the crowd, I could not identify one single adult that was not either significantly overweight or clinically obese. Worse yet, what really horrified me was the overwhelming prevalence of obesity in the children. I felt as though I had entered into the Twilight Zone. Although the entire scene seemed to evolve in slow motion before me, my mind was approaching light-speed overdrive as the future health implications of this phenomenon became obvious to me.

My heart sank as I viewed child after child, knowing what physical ailments would inevitably rob them of health, vitality, and perhaps even life, if they did not arrest this potentially lethal condition. I felt as though I was watching a very warped rendition of the TV program, "Bay Watch, " but instead of the beautiful shapely people, I was watching young boys so overweight that their pectorals boz.d with every step. This condition is referred to in medical terms as gynecomastia, or "female breasts," and it is indicative of many future health problems that will plague these young boys. Until that point I had not noticed how pandemic this problem had become. Staring at these children playing innocently, I thought to myself, "They are completely oblivious to the many psychological and medical problems they will be condemned to face in their future."

I looked toward the row of parents sitting in the lounge chairs watching their children play, and I thought, "Little do these children understand the enormous price they will have to pay tomorrow for this indiscretion in judgment from their parents today." How did it come to this? What has happened to America? Had I been asleep at the wheel for all these years? How can so many people sail blindly into this iceberg?

As a physician, I immediately began to think of the many negative health ramifications of this drastic change in our youth, not only for the present, but much more so for the future. A fearful thought immediately crossed my mind, "What will happen to the incidence of type 2 diabetes if this trend is not soon checked?" The increase of heart disease, stroke, arthritis, cancer and many psychological disorders, which may be directly or indirectly connected to obesity, will skyrocket in our nation. How will this affect our national healthcare system? The financial difficulty many are facing in these uncertain times will be compd.ed by the increase in the cost of healthcare. This will overwhelm an already stressed health insurance system that is already becoming too expensive for the average person to afford.

I was absolutely stunned, but my gears kept turning: "This is nothing less than a crime committed against these children, who do not have the capacity of understanding the negative ramifications of their obesity and the impact it will surely have in their future quality of life."

I looked toward the row of lounge chairs, with what must have been a puzzling look to anyone that was watching me, and asked myself, "Is it that parents don't care about the lethal ramifications obesity poses on their children? No… it must be that they are truly unaware of the serious damage they are doing to them. Don't they know that they are condemning them to a life filled with medical problems and potentially tragic and lethal consequences?"

At that moment, I felt my daughter's little hand squeezing mine. She looked up at me patiently, as if she knew I was somewhere in outer space and needed some time to land. My eyes locked unto her beautiful smile, and she knew I had landed. "Come on, Sarah, let's go see those slides," I said as I scooped her into my arms.

We had a blast those two days, but I could not get that gnawing thought out of my head. I came to the realization that if this trend is not reversed, the financial impact it will make in our nation will be astronomical. I resolved to look into the matter more thoroughly the first spare moment I had.

I have researched this extensively since that third epiphany at the indoor water park in Detroit. I am convinced that if a foreign power were to cause only half the damage to our people and to our economy that this trend will surely bring upon us, we would promptly declare war on them and immediately attack them with the entire arsenal of weapons at our disposal. Furthermore, if obesity and diabetes were infectious diseases that could be transmitted by an organism, I am convinced that public health officials and politicians would join ranks to promptly declare a state emergency of pandemic proportions.

Our nation is sailing into the "perfect storm," whose hurricane force winds will surely slam us against the iceberg and bring our ship to the bottom of the ocean, unless we change its course. The cost of healthcare will explode as insurance companies race to keep up with the exponentially rising expenses generated by the many diseases which will be spawned by this tragic increase in obesity.

This will inevitably have a significant impact in the wallet of every single person in our nation. Our nation's productivity will be diminished, as more of our population will become incapacitated by diseases directly or indirectly tied to this obesity, but the financial loss will be insignificant compared to the human loss. How many future children will lose their parents prematurely? "Someone needs to do something about this!" I thought. Then it struck me like a bolt of lightning: "I need to be that someone!"

For the sake of our children, we must begin to educate and mobilize our community in order to avert the coming crisis before the perfect storm comes together. And yet, the iceberg in our path remains obscured by the fog of ignorance as we sail headlong into a disaster of epic proportions.

Risks

The Age of Globesity

There are several factors that have contributed in synchrony to our present course. At the beginning of the twentieth century we entered into a new era in our nation, an era that was earmarked by shifts in our culture that were unprecedented in scope and magnitude throughout human history. The increasing amount and availability of food for the average person in our nation has truly transformed us into the "Land of Bounty."

The industrial revolution in the previous century had begun the process of the mechanization of farming methods. The motorized tractor, the use of commercial fertilizers, the ability to irrigate vast fields with motorized pumps, the use of modern pesticides, the development of modern farming techniques all combined to create a miraculous growth in the productivity of agricultural land. The fact that fewer people needed to work the land to provide food for the community allowed many more to migrate to the city and find other forms of employment. Although the conditions at first were dismal for city laborers, through collective bargaining our nation developed a middle class that had not been equaled by any other nation in the world before us.

None can ignore that the average person today works fewer hours than ever before in human history and has more "stuff" to show for his labor. For this same reason, more people than in any other nation ever before have access to more food than is required to survive. That is, the vast majority of our people in this nation have access to an overabundance of food. This economic boom has also given rise to an unprecedented access to cutting edge technology for the common man, which in times past was available only to the very wealthy class. Most homes now have two cars and a television set in every room. The washing machine and dryer have provided for the homemaker the opportunity to have much more leisure time than in times past. The strenuous nature of the work that was necessary to survive two hundred years ago has been replaced by modern conveniences, which allow us unprecedented levels of leisure time at our disposal.

Computers and television have made a huge impact on our culture. In the latter part of the twentieth century we entered the age of visual communication. We quickly traversed the line from auditory communication to visual communication with the inventions of the moving picture show, television, personal computers, satellites and the Internet. Through these marvels of technology we are literally connected with the entire planet from our personal homes. We have access to information at our fingertips that could not, in times past, be cataloged in the largest libraries of 99% of the cities in the world.

With all the wonderful advancements in technology and communications, we are now only beginning to understand the downside of these wonderful amenities. Instead of walking to our destinations, we drive while seated in cushioned chairs and air-conditioned vehicles. Many household chores that required physical exertion are now mechanically done for us. Electric household appliances have created awesome comforts for all of us but at the price of creating a more sedentary lifestyle for most people. As a matter of fact, most of us take the elevator to go up one floor.

In the not too distant past, most children spent the vast majority of their free time playing sports outside. When I was a child it took my mom close to an hour to chase me down and bring me home for dinner. If there was daylight I wanted to be outside, running and playing with my friends.

In stark contrast, today the vast majority of children lead a dangerously sedentary life, glued to the computer screen or television set. Only one in five children today participates in any physical after-school activities. Even more alarmingly, most of the schools are no longer providing physical education as part of their required curriculum. This disastrous trend in exercise deprivation is spiraling out of control, and the repercussions are very real and tangible in the future health of our people.

In 1982, only 4% of our children were overweight. By 2004 the number had more than quadrupled to a whopping 17.1%, and it is still rising. This problem is not exclusive to our children. Statistics show that over 25% of adults in the Unites States now live completely sedentary lifestyles and the majority of those who are not completely sedentary are borderline sedentary. This has created a growing problem (in more ways than one) that is catastrophic in scope. Two thirds of our adult population is now categorized as either clinically obese or overweight; not half…. two thirds!

Our lack of regular physical exercise is one of the key elements bringing us into alignment with that iceberg in the horizon, but it is not the only one. Here is the clincher: our sedentary lives are further complicated by the absolutely dismal choices we make in our diets. The fast-paced lifestyle of our culture has brought upon us the convenience of "fast foods." They are fast foods all right—foods that will quickly bring us to the grave.

Consider the typical meal of a ten-year-old child in a fast food chain restaurant. If he eats one double-cheeseburger with French fries and a 16-oz. soda pop he will ingest a total of approximately 860 calories, which is about 43% of his recommended daily caloric intake. This is if he does not get a refill, or an extra cheeseburger, or an ice cream sundae for desert. Not to mention that the high content of saturated fats will begin to line the arteries of this ten-year-old child with plaque that may one day kill him or her.

The use of sugar to stimulate sales in foods has created a maelstrom of health problems in our nation. And the sophistication of the advertisement campaigns to reach the minds of our children, in order to manipulate the parents through them, has become a true science, with marvelous financial rewards for the calloused and greedy merchants of our culture. Most parents are unaware that an 8-oz. glass of Coke contains 8 and ¾ spoons of sugar. Coke contains 12 calories per oz.. A Wendy's small drink contains 16 oz., or 192 calories. The medium drink is 20 oz., or 240 calories. The "biggie" contains 32 oz. (one quart), or 384 calories. But the big daddy of them all is the Big Gulp at 7-Eleven stores with 52 oz., which is a whopping 624 calories. This is 28% of the recommended daily calories for an adult man, and 35% for an adult woman--in just one drink!

The plain fact is that we are eating more than ever, eating the wrong types of foods, which are easily converted to fat, and not burning any calories with regular exercise. Americans spend nine times as many minutes watching television and movies as they do all other leisure activities combined. These three elements work synergistically to create the rising trend in clinical obesity that we are experiencing in our nation, and epidemic that is spreading around the globe as nations join our culture in the prevalence of fast foods, overconsumption, and lack of exercise. The rise in clinical obesity is being experienced by all the modern industrialized nations of the world, including China and India. We are now entering the Age of Globesity.

In America, the average caloric intake for a male has increased by 168 kcal/day in the last 30 years. The average caloric intake for women in our nation has increased by an astounding 335 kcal/day in the last 30 years. This by itself is extremely critical, but it is exponentially compd.ed by the high glycemic foods we now ignorantly consume.

That brings us to the fourth factor that is leading our nation to the coming perfect storm. Americans are for the most part unaware that some of the diets they are undertaking in order to lose weight are in fact causing them to gain weight. They are unaware of the danger of high glycemic carbohydrates. High glycemic foods are those that can be quickly converted to sugar by the body and subsequently stored as fat, as we shall later see.

Sadly, some who are attempting to eat correctly have been completely misguided by popular diet trends, which do not account for the high glycemic load found in many foods. These popular trends end up doing exactly the opposite of what they had hoped to produce. As a matter of fact, the typical American diet has increasingly become a dangerously high glycemic index diet.

We will deal with this more thoroughly later in this book, in order to equip the reader with the knowledge necessary to make the right choices in diet that can provide one with a better quality of life. But for now, I want to address the impact that this trend has made, and will make, in the health of our families, which is collectively impacting our nation in exponential numbers.

The Economic and Emotional Impact

The impact of globesity will inevitably spell financial ruin for our nation. The first and most powerful impact that this trend will produce is a dramatic rise in the incidence of diabetes in our population. There are two types of diabetes. Type 1 diabetes is typically detected during childhood and is seen in people who are genetically predisposed to the disease. Type 2 diabetes is not necessarily genetically linked. It usually has a late onset in adulthood and is directly linked to diet and obesity. Both type 1 and type 2 diabetes have disastrous effects upon our organs and create the same malevolent and disastrous health problems.

A recent study from the Centers for Disease Control and Prevention (CDC) co-authored by Jing Wang, MPH, and Edward W. Gregg, PhD, has concluded that every year since 1990 the incidence of type II diabetes has increased by 5% in America. In other words, today there are 90% more people suffering from the lethal and debilitating disease than in 1990, and the trend is not diminishing.

The American Diabetes Association highlights these CDC findings in Diabetes News. Linda S. Geiss, MA, Chief of Diabetes Surveillance, Diabetes Program, Division of Diabetes Translation, Centers for Disease Control and Prevention, stated, **"The growth in diabetes prevalence and incidence** accelerated in the early 1990's and this acceleration remains unabated...It is likely tied to the growth in obesity in this country, and if we are going to stem the growing burden of diabetes, we must improve our prevention efforts."

Today 23.6 million Americans, or 7.8% of the population, have diabetes. Even more alarming, 54 million Americans have pre-diabetes, an abnormally high level of elevated blood sugar, which is a pre-cursor to diabetes. Worse yet, some 6 million Americans do not even know that they have pre-diabetes because the disease has not yet become symptomatic enough. This means that almost one third of all Americans are now either diabetics or pre-diabetics, and many of them do not know it.

Today, the medical costs directly attributed to diabetes are a staggering 116 billion dollars per year. If we compute the associated costs of wages not earned and the lack of productivity due to absenteeism, the total cost to the economy is 174 billion dollars. If diabetes did not exist, in just a few years' time the savings would totally pay for our entire national debt. If this trend continues unchecked, it will be the perfect storm that shall surely sink our economy, not to mention the personal tragedies and heartaches that the disease will bring to millions of families. It is a burgeoning disaster of the first magnitude that can no longer be ignored.

The United States is not alone in this problem. As the nations of the world improve their economies and the standard of living increases, their time to fight the legendary "Midriff Dragon" and his faithful sidekick, "Diabetes," will also come. We are already seeing this escalating trend in the urban areas of India and China as the rising middle class begins to enjoy the luxuries of their increasing revenues.

US Diabetes Statistics
- *23.6 million diabetics*
- *54 million pre-diabetics*
- *6 million are unaware of pre-diabetic state*

We are now poised to stumble headlong into a new paradigm shift in our globe that will have severe health, financial, and psychological ramifications for every member of the human race. We are blindly entering into the "Age of Globesity," an age where obesity will become a global killer second to none.

But there is no need for doom and gloom! We can change this. I t is not written in stone. We can turn the ship around before entering the devastating hurricane winds of this perfect storm.... if we are willing.

In 1994, former United Sates Surgeon General C. Everett Koop founded an organization named *Shape Up America* as he became alarmed at the dramatic rise in the cases of diabetes in our nation. In order to bring a level of awareness to the link between obesity and diabetes, he coined the term "diabesity."

The dramatic rise in obesity is bringing with it a corresponding rise in diabetes. Hence, the term diabesity brings to us the awareness of this unholy wedlock between obesity and diabetes. The link has been further substantiated in the report made by the CDC, which examined weight trends among adults age 20 and over and found that obesity in the U.S. population began to increase more rapidly in 1986, four years prior to the time when diabetes began to increase significantly.

Obesity is the Midriff Dragon, and it is a major contributor to type 2 diabetes, which must be addressed if we hope to stem the alarming increase in the incidence of this terrible disease. The Midriff Dragon is the curse of affluence, but it need not be so. We can conquer this dreaded dragon that brings calamity and distress upon our planet. There is good reason to have hope, because 90% to 95% of all cases of diabetes are type 2. This means that we can make a significant impact on this disease if we are able to reverse the present trend in obesity, which is spreading throughout our planet in every age level, ethnic group, and gender like a raging firestorm.

We have no time to waste. Type 2 diabetes used to be called "late onset diabetes" because it was usually found in adults 40 years and older, as they became obese in late age. But as more children and adolescents are now becoming obese, the incidence of type 2 diabetes in children is increasing at a corresponding rate. Based on data acquired between 2002 and 2003, there were 18,700 youths newly diagnosed with type 1 and type 2 diabetes annually.

In 2007 there were 281,000 newly diagnosed cases of diabetes between the ages of 20 and 39 years old. There were 819,000 new cases of diabetes in the age bracket between 40 and 59 years old, and 536,000 in the age group 60 years old and upward. The total number of newly diagnosed cases of diabetes for 2007 amounted to 1,636,000 people in the United States alone.

Over one and one half million Americans every year are struck with a disease that will severely impair their quality of life and may lead to a premature death. What is most alarming is that this rate is escalating consistently by 5% every year. A recent study by the University of Chicago indicates that the number of Americans diagnosed with diabetes will double in the next 25 years, from 23.7 million in 2009. I fear that even this estimate is too low, if we are unable to change the factors leading to this disaster.

While it is true that modern medicine has enabled us to treat this disease, and those patients who keep to their prescribed treatment can fare relatively well, the most prudent action ought to be to prevent the disease and not to treat it after the fact. An oz. of prevention is truly worth more than one ton of cure.

Most people are simply not aware of the lethal nature or the serious consequences to our quality of life that this disease poses to all Americans. Even more frustrating to those of us who wish to sound the alarm are people who are apathetic, who do have some idea of the negative repercussions but simply shrug their shoulders and naively say, "This is something that happens to other people. It won't happen to me."

The plain fact is that obesity leads to diabetes, which leads to a host of other health problems, not the least of which is premature death.

The Link between Obesity and Morbidity

If you value being alive, then you may want to pay close attention to the following: According to the CDC, men diagnosed with diabetes by age forty will lose an average eleven years of their lifetime. Women in the same category will lose fourteen years of their lifetime.

Besides the diminished quality of life that many diabetics suffer during the years prior to their premature deaths, they are two to three times more likely to suffer from clinical depression. The incidence of depression in patients with diabetes is understandably high given the many difficulties they face.

Males with diabetes often have to deal with the emotional trauma of sexual impotence because of erectile dysfunction. An erection is triggered when the sensory information received by the nerve cells in the penis cause the blood vessels to become engorged, thus causing it to become erect. But when a man has diabetes it damages the nerves and they cannot communicate or transfer the nerve impulse to the penis. In addition, the poor circulation from inflamed blood vessels means that the penis cannot sustain adequate erection because of restricted blood flow. This sexual dysfunction becomes evident within ten years of the onset of high blood sugar. Over half of diabetic men 60 and older are impotent, but this also occurs in 9% of men inflicted by the disease even in their twenties.

Many patients experience a sense of doom and despair as they become aware of all of the negative physical complications that go hand-in-hand with the disease. The abrupt change in lifestyle that this disease brings upon its victims causes many psychological obstacles. A typical patient needs to regulate his life 24 hours a day and seven days a week for the rest of his life.

Those who like to live their lives spontaneously, with spur of the moment impulses, have the greatest difficulty adjusting. Spur of the moment lifestyles are gone forever for diabetics who wish to keep their blood sugar under control and avoid the physical repercussions of not doing so.

In some cases, the first sign of the disease may be one of the more severe complications. A patient may wake up one morning and find his vision blurred or darkened. Each year some 24,000 people in the United States go blind because of diabetes. It is the leading cause of blindness in our nation. Most of the time these severe complications are the result of prolonged noncompliance with the prescribed regimens that keep blood sugar levels within normal limits.

In 2004, 71,000 people had a non-traumatic amputation of some kind due to diabetes. The decrease in circulation which accompanies this disease can sometimes lead to gangrene, causing many to undergo amputations of toes, feet and even their legs. More than 60% of lower limb amputations done in the United States are due to diabetes.

Poorly controlled type I diabetes before conception and during the first trimester of pregnancy results in major birth defects in 5-10% of cases and spontaneous abortions in 15-20% of cases. Expectant mothers who are overweight run the risk of developing type 2 diabetes. These women need careful monitoring by the physician and sometimes even require insulin injections. Gestational diabetes usually goes away after birth, but the mother then has a two-in-three chance that it will return in future pregnancies; some women with gestational diabetes will eventually develop type 2 diabetes permanently.

Each year 28,000 people end up with kidney failure because of diabetes. It is the leading cause of kidney failure in the United States. In 2005 a total of 178,689 people with end-stage kidney disease due to diabetes were living on chronic dialysis or with a kidney transplant. Those who are healthy or fortunate enough to find a match may have a kidney transplant. Those less fortunate are condemned to the regular use of the dialysis machine to stay alive. Once a week, and sometimes more often, they must go through the arduous dialysis procedure in order to stay alive. The stress that the machine places on the heart adds another danger to the already difficult equation.

Diabetes damages arteries and organs and destroys the cells in the human body. In 2004, heart disease was noted on 68% of the death certificates of individuals 65 and older with diabetes-related. In that same year and category, 16% of them had suffered strokes. Diabetics have a two to four times higher death rate by heart disease and two to four times higher risk of stroke than non-diabetic individuals. Plainly stated, diabetes leads to arteriosclerosis, strokes and heart attacks, as we shall later address more completely.

The bottom line is that diabetes is the seventh leading killer in the United States and was directly responsible for 72,507 deaths in 2006. However, this ranking is based on death certificate reports in which diabetes was listed as the primary cause of death. Realistically, this number is not an accurate description of the true lethality of this disease. If we consider the number of death certificates where diabetes was listed as a contributor to the death, the number of deaths was 233,619 in 2005, the latest year for which data was available at the time this book was being written.

Even this figure may be hopelessly unrealistic. The National Diabetes Statistics, where these figures are posted, notes, "Diabetes is likely to be underreported as a cause of death. Studies have found that only about 35 to 40 percent of decedents with diabetes had it listed anywhere on the death certificate and only about 10 to 15 percent had it listed as the underlying cause." (National Diabetes Information Clearinghouse (NDIC), *National Diabetes Statistics 2007*, Pg. 7)

If we assume the most conservative estimate from NDIC of 40%, this means that the actual number of deaths that are at least partially contributable to diabetes is 588,047 annually. If we assume the 35% figure then the number of annual deaths that are directly or indirectly attributable to diabetes is around 667,482.

This number represents more than 13 times as many American victims each year from diabetes as in the entire Vietnam War.

More than half a million people are directly or indirectly killed each year by this disease and the numbers continue to climb. Unless we as a nation begin to address this rising storm, the number of fatalities will continue to rise meteorically. We will not have to wait long before this statistic becomes more than just a number, before someone in our immediate family is struck down before their time.

In an article titled "New Survey Results Show Huge Burden of Diabetes," in the National Institute of Health News (NIH News) published by the U. S. Department of Health and Human Services, the alarm was sounded.

"We're facing a diabetes epidemic that shows no signs of abating, judging from the number of individuals with pre-diabetes," said lead author Catherine Cowie, PhD, of the National Institute of Diabetes and Digestive and Kidney Diseases (NIDDK), a part of the National Institutes of Health (NIH). "For years, diabetes prevalence estimates have been based mainly on data that included a fasting glucose test but not an OGTT [oral glucose tolerance test]. The 2005-2006 National Health and Nutrition Examination Survey, or NHANES, is the first national survey in 15 years to include the OGTT. The addition of the OGTT gives us greater confidence that we're seeing the true burden of diabetes and pre-diabetes in a representative sample of the U.S. population." (*NIH News*, January 26, 2009)

Four factors working synergistically are combining to form the perfect storm, which may destabilize our nation and wreak havoc on our families. These are:

1. Chronic physical deprivation. Regular exercise is essential to burn calories that the body would otherwise store as fat and also to establish a healthy musculoskeletal system to protect joints and increase vitality.

2. Dependency on fast foods that facilitate hectic lifestyles.

3. Consumption of high glycemic diets (foods that easily elevate blood sugar levels), even by those attempting to eat right.

4. Habitual overconsumption (gluttony).

Each of these contributing factors must be adequately addressed in order to dismantle the basic components that if left untreated will produce the coming cataclysm of our generation.

Having said all that, the amount that we eat is very important. I f we do not restrict the amount of calories we ingest below the level that the body uses, we will gain weight no matter what diet we are on. For this reason it is also absolutely imperative that we exercise to burn the calories we consume and keep the glucose and subsequently the insulin level in our blood within the proper levels.

All of us expend energy every moment that we are alive, even when we sleep. As our body uses the energy that we have ingested to do the many varied chemical processes that our body needs to live, we burn the calories that we have ingested. The resting energy expenditure of the average adult is known as the basal metabolic rate (BMR). This amounts to about 10-12 calories per pd. of body weight every day. Although the rate may vary slightly from person to person other, it averages 1,400 calories per day. This is what we need minimally to simply stay alive in a resting state. When we get up from our beds and move around in our daily routines, we increase the number of calories that we burn. The average adult man has a daily energy expenditure of about 2, 300 calories, and the average adult woman has a daily expenditure of about 1,800 to 2,000 calories.

The more physical exertion we do, the more calories we burn. Therefore, if our caloric intake is not balanced by our caloric output we store the excess calories in the form of fat and glycogen, as we shall see. Hence, our diet plan must include a certain amount of daily exercise if we hope to effectively reduce or control our weight. For this reason, the present trend in public school systems to eliminate physical education must be addressed beginning at the local levels. Parents must take this charge, not waiting for politicians to act judiciously. Pressure must be placed upon our school boards to do away such items as soft drinks, which are disastrous to our children in the school cafeterias. If we hope to stem the tide, we must reeducate our educators to promote balanced healthy diets with a low glycemic index.

How it Works

The Importance of the Glycemic Index

What is the glycemic index? In order to understand the dangerous physical repercussions of diets that can lead us into diabetes, we must first understand the concept of the glycemic index. We must also understand the role that insulin plays in regulating sugar in our bodies. These topics are a bit technical, but our understanding of this process is crucial if we are to make truly informed choices in this matter of life and death, literally. I will try to make it as simple as possible to understand.

The glycemic index is a tool that allows us to measure how quickly foods turn into sugar in our blood after being ingested. As it turns out, this index has significant health ramifications in many areas, not the least of which is that it shows us which foods will cause an undesirable insulin spike in our blood. However, before we discuss this process, let us first understand a little about how our body works and how the foods that we ingest affect it.

There are three main elements in our food that are essential to our bodies. These are fatty acids (fats), proteins, and carbohydrates. Each of these has a unique function in the metabolism of our bodies. If we are to remain in optimum health, then ingesting the right proportions of these elements is absolutely imperative.

Most of us have heard that high-fat diets are dangerous to our health, but few of us understand that diets without fat but with a high glycemic index will cause excess calories to be converted to and stored as fat within our bodies.

Eating low fat diets, but with carbohydrates that have a high glycemic index, will still result in the overproduction and storage of fat in our bodies.

A certain amount of fat is necessary for our cells to be able to manufacture the chemicals that are necessary for the body to function properly. Without fats the body will fail to produce essential hormones and digestive acids, but too much fat will trigger a host of chemical reactions that are extremely harmful to our health, as we shall later see.

Fats are used to store energy and to produce certain hormones and digestive acids. They are also essential for the lubrication of joints and for maintaining healthy skin. If a woman becomes too thin due to an eating disorder, famine, illness, or even some extreme physical training, she may stop menstruating because she cannot produce the hormones she needs to menstruate without fats.

The right amount of fat is essential to optimum health. On the other hand, if a woman has excess fat she may produce excess estrogen. For this reason, obesity is also linked with breast cancer. In men, obesity may inhibit the production of androgens (male hormones), which will in turn reduce libido, and it may further increase the production of estrogen, causing gynecomastia (female breasts in men). A higher than normal level of estrogen in men has also been linked to cancer.

Proteins are made up of long chains of amino acids, which the body rips apart and recombines to make the many different kinds of proteins our cells need to function. Amino acids are like letters in an alphabet that when put together in unique sequences can create a specific word, or protein. Each protein is used for a specific task. They are the building blocks of life. The body transforms them into muscle, hormones, and other chemicals required for cell function in our bodies. Our diets must therefore contain a certain amount of foods that contain proteins.

Carbohydrates produce the fuel necessary for our cells to do work. Our body breaks down the carbohydrates into glucose, which is the fuel that energizes our metabolic functions. Without this fuel, the proteins cannot be taken apart and reconstructed in the many kinds necessary for life to exist. This sugar (glucose) is our body's fuel, and just like our cars, without fuel our motor can't run. Carbohydrates are essential for the brain and for red blood cells, and they are also the main source of fuel for the muscles when exercising strenuously.

In the past, the terms used to classify carbohydrates were "simple carbohydrates," and "complex carbohydrates." Carbohydrates were described by the nature of their molecular structures. Small molecules, like sugars, were labeled as simple carbohydrates. Carbohydrates with larger molecular structures, like starches, were referred to as complex carbohydrates. It was assumed that by virtue of their larger size they would be slowly digested and absorbed gradually into the bloodstream. This is desirable because the elevation of our blood sugar would then be also slower, avoiding the insulin spikes in our bloodstream. Insulin rises step by step as the glucose in our blood rises.

For many years we believed that eating complex carbohydrates was better than simple carbohydrates. This was taught as an absolute fact for fifty years in medical schools, but it turns out not to be true.

Many "complex carbohydrates" can be absorbed quickly into the blood stream, thus elevating our blood sugar rapidly. This quick rise in the blood sugar levels then causes a spike in the insulin production. Also, some "simple carbohydrates" can be absorbed more gradually into our blood stream, creating a more gradual rise in the level of glucose in our blood. We have discovered that the rise in the level of glucose in our blood cannot be predicted simply on the basis of the size of the molecular structure of the carbohydrates.

Scientists were completely surprised when "complex carbohydrates" such as bread, potatoes, and rice were quickly absorbed and significantly raised blood glucose levels rather rapidly. Most of the sugars contained in other carbohydrate foods, on the other hand, produced a more moderate rise in blood-glucose than most starches. These terms have therefore been recently discarded, when it was discovered that the classifications were basically scientifically meaningless and inadequate in creating a comparative analysis of the individual foods.

In its place we have instituted the glycemic index, which measures how rapidly each carbohydrate elevates our blood sugar level. To be more specific, it measures the real metabolic reaction of the food in the body, in that it graphs the amount of glucose that is carried by the blood after the ingestion of a particular carbohydrate within a given amount of time. The numbers are measured against a standard that provides for a relative grouping of the specific food items. In other words, the glycemic index uses a numbering system that compares each food item to the standard of pure glucose, which therefore allows us to determine a realistic comparison between the different carbohydrates that grades how each of them affect our blood glucose levels.

By measuring the effect of all the different carbohydrates known to mankind, we are able to then establish a glycemic index that allows us to determine how much and how rapidly our blood glucose level will rise after ingesting each of these items. Using the glycemic index, we can keep the amount of insulin produced in our body within its proper level by avoiding the consumption of the carbohydrates with a high glycemic value, so that it will not have the undesirable repercussions we wish to prevent, as we shall see.

This breakthrough was pioneered by Dr. David Jenkins, a professor of nutrition, and Tom Wolever, along with other colleagues at the University of Toronto, the same university where insulin had been discovered in 1921. They were the first to introduce the term "glycemic index," as they investigated how foods behaved in the bodies of real people.

Traditionalists initially hotly debated the revolutionary findings, which seemed to them to be counterintuitive. The proponents and opponents almost came to blows in many conferences aimed at finding a consensus. Today, almost three decades later, the evidence is indisputable. The glycemic index has become a clinically proven tool in the treatment of diabetics, weight control, and coronary health after countless scientific studies in the United Kingdom, France, Italy, Sweden, Australia and Canada. However, old paradigms die hard and the United States remains officially opposed.

The resulting confusion has led many Americans to adopt low-fat diets that are dangerously deceptive because they do not take into account the glycemic index and can therefore lead to obesity and diabetes, rather than health.

1.1 – How the Glycemic Index (GI) is Derived

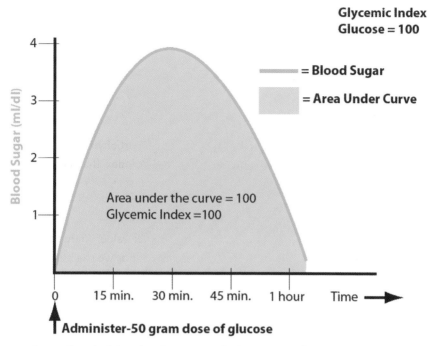

Administer-50 gram dose of glucose

By orally administering 50 grams of glucose to a fasting patient, we are able to follow the blood sugar levels following its ingestion.

As you can see, following the green line, there is a very rapid rise in blood sugar soon after ingesting the 50 gm. dose, resulting in a high peak, which then quickly drops. By arbitrarily assigning the number 100 to correspond with the area under the curve (shaded light green), we can then begin an index, or standard, which we can use to compare different carbohydrate foods.

By repeating this sequence with each of the carbohydrate foods, we wish to measure, we can come up with a relative number that can be compared to the standard of pure glucose. For example, instead of giving the fasting patient a dose of 50 grams of glucose, we give him 50 grams of cherries. We then trace the blood sugar levels through time, and by calculating the area under the curve we establish a relative number called the glycemic index value for cherries, which is 22.

1.2 – GI of Cherries

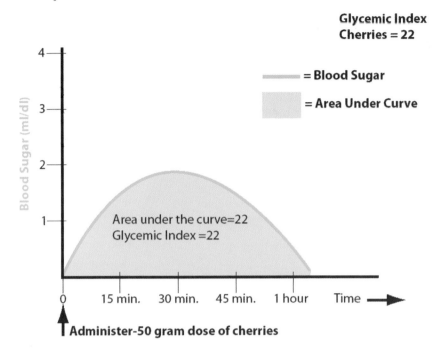

**Glycemic Index
Cherries = 22**

━━━━ **= Blood Sugar**

▨ **= Area Under Curve**

Area under the curve=22
Glycemic Index =22

0   15 min.   30 min.   45 min.   1 hour   Time ➔

Administer-50 gram dose of cherries

The Glycemic Load

The use of the glycemic load is an essential tool in determining the quantity of carbohydrates our body needs. The glycemic index is a tool that allows us to measure the quality of a particular carbohydrate. We are able to observe that diets with carbohydrates having low glycemic index values will not create the adverse physical repercussions that lead to morbid obesity and diabetes.

Conversely, those diets which contain carbohydrates with high glycemic index values will lead us into that dangerous mine field. However, the quality of the carbohydrate will become a moot point if the quantities ingested are beyond the normal spectrum necessary for the body to function at optimum health.

Researchers at Harvard University coined the term "glycemic load" in order to establish a system that would account for the overall quantity of the carbohydrates ingested in a meal. While the glycemic index measures the quality, the glycemic load computes the overall quantity of the carbohydrates ingested. It is a tool that measures the quantity, while yet acknowledging the quality factor as well.

This is calculated by multiplying the glycemic index (quality) by the amount of the available carbohydrate (quantity) ingested for that serving. This number is then divided by 100 and the result is the glycemic load.

For example, parboiled rice has a glycemic index of 72. A nominal portion would be around 1 cup. Multiplying the glycemic index of 72 by the portion of one cup of rice (which has 36 grams of available carbohydrates) we would come up with 72 x 36 = 2592. We then divide 2592 by 100 and we arrive at the glycemic load of 26, just for the rice (2592/100 = 25.92, rounded to 26).

If we add another carbohydrate to that meal, we must follow the same procedure and add the two glycemic loads together. Hence, if we add to this meal another carbohydrate such as butter beans, whose glycemic index is 28, with a portion of 150 grams (which gives us 20 grams of available carbohydrates), then we come to the number 28 x 20= 560. Dividing 560 by 100, we come to the glycemic load of this portion of butter beans (560/100 = 5.6, rounded to 6).

Adding the glycemic load of rice with the glycemic load of the butter beans, we get 26 + 6 = 32. This is the glycemic load for that meal.

If we want to lose weight, then we should try to use carbohydrates whose glycemic index is less than 55. Once we come to the end of the day and we add together the glycemic loads of all foods eaten, the total number of that day's glycemic load should be below 140. This means that our weekly glycemic load should be less than 980 (140 x 7 = 980).

If we are not interested in losing weight, but only in maintaining, then we can shoot for a cumulative daily glycemic load that is below 160. Our weekly glycemic load should then be below 1120 (160 x 7 = 1120). However, we must understand that using carbohydrates of a glycemic index value that is greater than 55 will create insulin spikes, which are detrimental to our optimum health, as we earlier described.

In moderation, our body can absorb these occasional exceptions to our goal, but if we make a habit of splurging one day and then trying to overcome it with other days of ingesting very low glycemic index foods, we defeat our purpose of maintaining optimum health. Such a disastrous habit will only lead to the eventual exhaustion of the beta cells that produce the insulin.

The glycemic load by itself is therefore not exclusively indicative of the diet that we must attain to reach optimum health and avoid the pitfalls of obesity and diabetes. We must attempt to choose the carbohydrates that have a glycemic index below 55 as much as possible if we hope to keep our poor beta cells from collapsing from exhaustion and quitting their vital job.

The glycemic load helps us to determine if we are eating too much. Quantity is important if we wish to avoid turning the energy from these carbohydrates into fat within our bodies. If we ingest more than our body can use we store the excess in fat. Some of us have a very real problem with overeating. The psychological factors contributing to this problem are numerous.

Conquering the Midriff Dragon – Low Fat Diets vs. Low Carb Diets

The dramatic rise in cardiovascular disease in our nation at the end of the twentieth century sparked an interest in low fat diets, as physicians hoped to stem the alarming tide of increase arteriosclerosis and the attending cardiovascular problems it creates. These low fat diets were naturally high in carbohydrates, but the real differences between the various carbohydrates were not well appreciated at that time. Many who consumed carbohydrates with a high glycemic index would in the end continue to store fats rather than lose weight. Moreover, all kinds of fat were vilified and most of us were taught to avoid it like the plague.

The truth is that our bodies need a balance of carbohydrates, proteins, and fats to function properly. But just like all carbohydrates are not equal, so all fats are not equal either. Saturated fats, which tend to be in solid form at room temperature, are very harmful because they clog arteries and contribute to the formation of plaque, the arteriosclerosis that causes coronary heart disease.

Saturated fats, including hydrogenated vegetable oil, shortening, and butter that are commonly used to fry foods in restaurants, are quite dangerous to our health. The fat in fatty meats and dairy products are also saturated fats.

However, the fats in fish, lean meats, olive oil, safflower oil, sunflower oil, and canola oil are unsaturated fat. These are actually necessary to properly maintain optimum health.

In the past, all fats were improperly lumped together as foods to be avoided. Even the most essential of fats, the polyunsaturated fats, were incorrectly avoided. These long-chain fats are fundamental to optimum human health. Research has shown that unsaturated fats such as those contained in olive oil, which are rich in Omega 3 and Omega 9, are actually indispensable in reducing the inflammation that leads to arteriosclerosis in our arteries.

More recently the Atkins Diet has challenged the proponents of the low fat diets with a revolutionary alternative. Initially, many physicians opposed it fearing that the low carbohydrate diets, which have a much higher percentage of fat in them, would increase cardiovascular risk. But research has shown the opposite. People who correctly followed the Atkins regimen have typically reduced their blood cholesterol and triglycerides and the risk factors associated with them.

How can a diet that is high in fat cause the reduction of fat in our bodies? It seems completely contrary to logic, but when properly followed the low carbohydrate diet reduces the amount of insulin that is secreted into the bloodstream because there is little intake of foods that can be rapidly produced into glucose. It is the rise of glucose in the blood that triggers the production of insulin. As it turns out, this reduction in the level of insulin results in less insulin resistance created in the cells, less fat storage, less glycogen storage, and less hunger. Moreover, when there is no glucose intake, then the body resorts to our fat stores as the source of energy and therefore reduces our visceral fat (the midriff bulge) as an alternative source of fuel. In other words, if we do not ingest carbohydrates our body will use the stored fat as fuel and we will lose weight. However, there are some problems with this extreme method that we must later address.

Time has shown that the traditional thinking that sought to encourage diets containing large percentages of carbohydrates, while avoiding fats and allowing only for small portions of meats (proteins), had limited success in reducing blood cholesterol or triglyceride levels and relied on strict calorie counting measures to successfully lose weight. These contained several flaws, as we shall see.

Ultimately, we must consider that the effectiveness of a diet is weighed by several factors. Reason and our newest scientific knowledge leads us to eight rules that lead to a healthy diet.

1. The diet must be maintainable for the long term, or it will result in the discouraging seesaw effect that inevitably demoralizes the dieter. It must be viewed as a permanent change in lifestyle and not as a fad or temporary change in eating habits for a limited period of time. This form of dieting is a recipe only for disaster and frustration. As a matter of fact, seesaw weight fluctuations can produce other health risks.

2. In order to be maintainable, the diet must therefore include enough variety to keep the person from tiring of the foods. If the foods ingested in a diet are not palatable the dieter will soon abandon the regimen.

3. The diet must balance all three categories (proteins, carbohydrates and fats) in such a way as to provide basic metabolic raw materials in the needed proportions to maximize health. Remember, our body needs all three components.

4. The diet must include foods that can provide for a variety of micronutrients that our bodies need to have optimum health. Therefore, it cannot be too exclusive in the variety of the foods, or many essential micronutrients will be sacrificed.

5. The diet must avoid:

    a. High glycemic index carbohydrates, which will produce insulin spikes that will counter weight loss efforts by kicking into gear the fat storing mechanism in the body.

    b. Saturated fats and trans-saturated fats, which are associated with an increase in cardiovascular disease.

6. The diet must include a physical regimen that is realistic for the individual, and the portions of ingested food must not exceed in total calories one's individual daily caloric output.

7. The diet must include foods with enough roughage to aid in the elimination process in order to avoid a host of medical problems.

8. Finally, it must be uncomplicated enough to be followed by the average person. Most people simply do not have the discipline or the

patience to measure and weigh every portion of their foods, and count the calories before eating.

Unfortunately, many of the low fat diets, which are supposed to prevent the introduction of fat into our system, are in fact producing dangerous levels of fat in the unwary dieter, because they contain carbohydrate foods with high glycemic indexes. These foods with high glycemic index not only create dangerous spikes in the insulin blood levels, with disastrous physical consequences, but also in the end they turn to fat in our bodies, adding to our visceral fat and the dangerous health complications created by the Midriff Dragon.

More importantly, few of us understand that an excess of insulin in our bodies is many times more harmful to our overall health than fat itself. The overabundance of insulin in our blood is the most dangerous culprit, wreaking havoc to our organs. A high insulin level in our blood is the principle cause of obesity and ultimately type 2 diabetes because it stimulates the storage of fat and exhausts the beta cells in our pancreas, where the insulin is made.

The overabundance of fat is also quite harmful in a variety of ways. Fat can be found in our bodies in two main areas, under our skin and in the core of the body. Subcutaneous fat (fat under our skin) serves as insulation and cushion to our bodies. Too much subcutaneous fat is called cellulite, the bumpy fat on our thighs and rear ends which all of us detest.

Although cellulite is not very appealing, it is not as harmful as the visceral fat in the core of our bodies, or being carrying excess weight in the middle abdominal region. The visceral fat is the Midriff Dragon, and people with visceral fat, or wide mid-girth, are much more at risk for diabetes and cardiovascular disease than those who have normal mid-girths. The Midriff Dragon is rarely far from his sidekick Diabetes.

Visceral fat is metabolically more active and creates **adipocytes**, which pick up the extra glucose, fatty acids, and amino acids in our bloodstream after we eat and convert them into even more stored fat. These adipocytes are like busy little squirrels picking up many kinds of nuts and storing them in a chest for winter in the form of fat cells. Unfortunately, when the treasure trove of nuts reaches a certain breaking point, the treasure chest begins to leak out the nuts. When our fat cells become "overstuffed" they have a tendency to leak fat molecules into the surrounding tissue and organs. For this reason, visceral fat near the core of our bodies is more dangerous as it is closer to many of our vital organs. This leakage of fat into our organs creates a host of pathological problems.

When fat gets inside muscle cells it interferes with their ability to respond to insulin. Insulin is the hormone "key" that opens the "door" in our cells to allow the glucose (fuel) to enter. It is created in the beta cells found in our pancreas. When fat "leaks" into our muscle cells, the muscle will not take up the fuel (glucose) it needs to work efficiently. Therefore, the body responds by making more insulin to send to the muscle, thinking that there is not enough in the blood. The beta cells crank up more insulin into the blood, creating an even higher spike. But, after some time, the beta cells become exhausted and cannot keep up with the continuous demand and the production of insulin begins to decline. If the process goes uncorrected for a given period of time, the patient develops type II diabetes as the beta cells quit working properly.

Simply stated, fat creates many serious problems to our organs. If fat goes into our muscle cells it interferes with the insulin that allows glucose to enter and be used as fuel in our muscles. If fat goes inside the pancreas it interferes with its ability to create insulin. Additionally, if fat goes inside the liver it interferes with the liver's capacity to respond to the insulin.

When our cells have been exposed to high levels of insulin in our blood for a given period of time, they become insulin resistant. Insulin resistance creates a further demand on the beta cells to produce more insulin, until the busy little beta cells become exhausted and can no longer function properly.

Hence, visceral fat is an essential culprit in the process of developing type 2 Diabetes. Obesity is a sure track to disaster in our future. If we hope to conquer the Midriff Dragon, we must therefore learn how to penetrate the dragon scales with our sword. If we do not take the time and effort to learn the art of dragon killing, the dragon will kill us.

We must bring to the battle the weapons that will rid us of the Midriff Dragon. It is my opinion that one of the most crucial weapons in our arsenal is the glycemic index, which can help us to eat the right carbohydrates that will not easily turn to fat and subsequently create all the cascading negative physiological disorders associated with high levels of fat and the over-production of insulin.

The following chart (Fig. 2.1) has listed a number of common carbohydrate foods with their glycemic index values. Those with a high glycemic index should be avoided in order to reduce spikes in insulin. This will reduce the total amount of insulin our body produces and subsequently the amount of fat our body stores.

2.1 - Limited Glycemic Index Table*
Low GI - 55 or below | Medium GI - 56 to 65 | **High GI - 65 or above**

Glucose- 100	Raisins- 64	Quaker Puffed Wheat- 67
Maltose- 105	Baked Potato- 85	Kellogg's Rice Crisps - 82
Sucrose- 65	Pretzels- 81	Broccoli- 15
Lactose- 46	Dates- 103	Asparagus- 15
Fructose- 23	Grapefruit- 25	Artichoke- 15
Baguettes- 95	Rice cakes- 77	Celery- 15
White Bread - 71	Doughnut- 76	Cauliflower- 15
White Rolls- 73	Waffles- 76	Cucumber- 15
Ezekiel Bread- 36	Peanuts- 14	Tomatoes- 15
Taco Shells- 68	Cashews- 22	Green Beans- 15
Cherries- 22	Whole Milk- 22	Lettuce - 15
Apples- 38	Skim Milk- 32	Zucchini- 15
Pears- 38	Oatmeal- 49	Peppers- 15
Peaches- 42	Graham Crackers- 74	Chickpeas- 33
Oranges- 44	Melba Toast- 70	Kidney Beans- 29
Pineapple- 66	Kellogg's Corn Flks.- 84	Pop Corn- 55
Watermelon- 72	Shredded Wheat- 67	Corn Chips- 74

* Limited sample. For a more complete list of the glycemic index see the **Appendix - Glycemic Index and Glycemic Load***s charts in the back of the book.*

The glycemic index is useful to us in another way, because it allows us to track the level of insulin created by these specific food items. If we consume foods that have a high glycemic index we create a corresponding high spike in insulin, which leads to the problems we have already discussed.

If we were to graph the insulin levels in the blood, in the same graph that we chart the glucose levels, we would find that the up-slope of the insulin chart mirrors the up-slope of the glucose chart almost step by step. Therefore, foods containing a high glycemic index number also produce high levels of insulin in our bodies.

In the following chart (Fig. 2.2) we can see that properly working beta cells will keep up with the rise in blood glucose. But notice that as time goes by, the glucose begins to drop while the insulin remains high within our blood.

As the insulin opens the door of our cells, the glucose is ushered inside and used as fuel. After some time, the fuel is consumed and yet the insulin remains in the bloodstream. This is bad.

2.2 - Insulin Levels After Ingesting High GI Carbohydrates

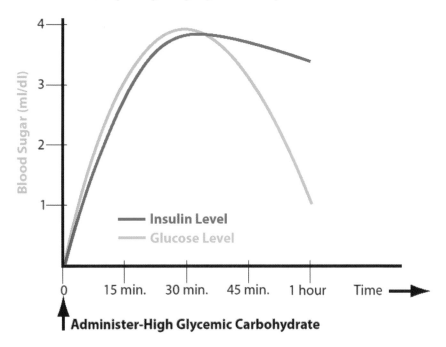

On the other hand, as we can see in Fig. 2.3, foods having a low glycemic index reduce the amount of insulin created by the beta cells and prevent the many negative side effects attending insulin spikes in our blood.

As time goes by, the use of the fuel (glucose) by our cells eventually lowers the amount of glucose in our blood, but notice that the amount of insulin is also diminished in this scenario. This not only spares the beta cells from the furious pace of overproducing insulin, but it keeps the amount of insulin in our blood at a low level and thus avoids the problem of insulin resistance.

If we consciously choose to consume foods from the glycemic index charts that have a low glycemic index, we can therefore strike at the heart of the Midriff Dragon with our lethal sword.

But, if we consume foods that have a high glycemic index, we shall instead feed the Midriff Dragon until he is large enough to kill us.

2.3 - Insulin Level After Ingesting Low GI Carbohydrates

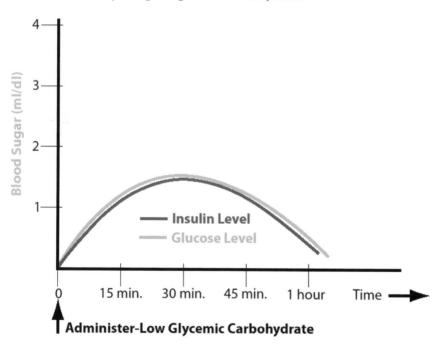

Our Two Fuel Tanks

Our body is consuming energy from the first moment of our life until the day we die. Since we are not eating continuously, our body must store energy so that it can be released when the need arises. This is accomplished through our liver by storing glycogen. The average adult person carries about two pd. of glycogen, which converts to about 4,000 calories. For every pd. of glycogen stored in our body, there is also the addition of approximately two pd. of water that is essential to the conversion process. As we use the glycogen, we excrete the water associated with the metabolic process as urine.

The liver is our primary fuel tank. In the following chart we can see that the glucose in the liver is our preferred fuel, since it provides quick energy for immediate use.

3.1 - The liver is our primary fuel tank, providing quick energy in the form of glycogen. Glycogen is a long chain of glucose (sugar) molecules.

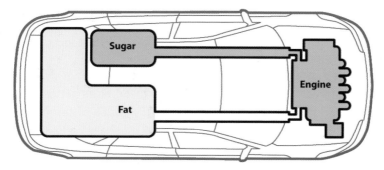

The second way that our body stores energy is by converting the foods we eat into fat. This secondary fuel tank provides a backup system should we not have food available so that our metabolic processes could continue to operate without interruption.

When we eat carbohydrates, our body converts this food into glycogen. But if we go on a low carbohydrate diet, our body chooses to leave a minimal amount of what fuel we have stored as glycogen in the liver and instead turns to the use of fat as a fuel. In other words, as our glycogen stores become diminished our body switches to fat as its primary source of energy. At this point, fat is broken down and released as fatty acids that may be converted into ketones. The muscle tissue has no problem using fat as a fuel, but the brain and the nervous system do. These ketones can be used for providing energy in the brain and the nervous system but not with the same efficiency as glycogen. The reliance on ketones as a fuel usually results in some weakness and fatigue, because the process is not designed to give quick bursts of energy, but rather to maintain the motor working during times of famine.

3.2 - This is the body's 2nd tank. It is designed to provide long lasting energy.

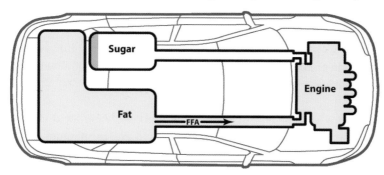

This form of metabolism has a side benefit in that it also reduces our hunger. In addition, by switching to our visceral fat rather than the glycogen stored in our liver as our source of energy there is a more rapid loss of body weight, which targets the dangerous visceral excess fat. Concurrently, this reduction of glucose in the blood also produces a marked reduction in insulin resistance.

These stored fats are, in fact, designed to be an important factor in regulating the fuel levels in our blood during the period of fasting between meals under normal circumstances. But they are especially useful to us during times of food scarcity, in order to maintain metabolic functions when there is little caloric intake. Throughout most of human history, scarcity has been the rule and not the exception. This incredible back-up fuel system enables us to endure periods of famines that would otherwise have killed us.

Most of us think that our visceral fat comes only from eating fatty foods and excesses of protein, but fats also come from the consumption of carbohydrates with high glycemic indexes, which cause insulin spikes in our blood. This insulin spike stimulates the conversion of the sugar in our blood to fat by the adipose cells. As insulin comes in contact with our fat cells (adipose tissue) it modifies them so that they become more active in breaking down, taking up, and storing fats that we have consumed. High levels of insulin therefore cause high levels of stored fat.

The storage of a moderate amount of fat is a necessary function of the body to protect itself against a metabolic imbalance during long fasts between meals. We can look at the fat cells as a second reserve tank in our bodies that is used for long trips that require long-range capabilities.

Some of us are genetically predisposed to store more fat than others. In an environment of scarce food, as in most of human history, this would be a decided advantage, allowing person to have greater reserves of fuel. The much greater need of physical exertion for survival in our past history favored those who had a better ability to survive during times of famine. However, in our modern world of abundance and low physical requirements, it now becomes a decided handicap.

The majority of us are no longer required to do heavy labor in our daily routines. Therefore, it is important that we plan to exercise in order to keep us from building excess fat. Although there are some genetic elements to obesity and diabetes, all of these can be countered through the right behavioral choices, as we shall further discuss.

Unfortunately for modern industrialized man, an excess of blood glucose will result in the excess production of fat that will not be used during the physical activity of the individual between meals in our present sedentary lifestyles. Our reserve tank then becomes too bulky for our car, and instead of helping us it begins to become a lethal liability.

The lack of exercise, which keeps us from burning the calories stored in the fat, and the overabundance of high glycemic carbohydrates in our typical modern diets, naturally result in the storage of even more fat. This process then will inevitably lead to obesity. Each pd. of fat represents an excess of 3,500 calories that we consumed but did not use.

The glycogen in the liver is used for quick bursts of energy, but it does not have the long lasting ability to fuel us that fat does. The energy stored in one gram of fat far exceeds that stored in one gram of starch. This stored energy is necessary for prolonged activity and can therefore only be burned through prolonged physical activity, when elevated levels of glucose and insulin are not present in our blood. This is important in choosing the kind of exercises we are to do, if we hope to burn the fat and not just the glycogen reserves in the liver.

Intense exercises for short periods of time rely on the burning of glycogen. Prolonged exercises of even a more moderate nature will, on the other hand, begin to activate the second fuel tank and will help us to burn the visceral fat as fuel.

When we deplete our glucose fuel through prolonged exercise or even with normal metabolism when our carbohydrate intake consists of low glycemic foods, the body then converts fat into free fatty acids, which are used as the alternate fuel source (the second tank).

3.3 - The conversion of fat into free fatty acids can be used as fuel.

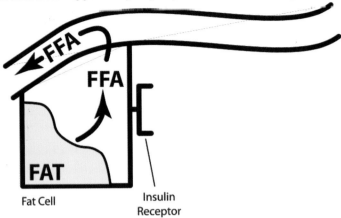

Fat Cell

Insulin
Receptor

FFA = Free Fatty Acid

However this conversion of fat into free fatty acids that can be used for fuel can only take place when both the bloods sugar is low and the insulin level is also low. This is achieved when we consume carbohydrates with a low glycemic index.

3.4 - The conversion of fats to free fatty acids can only occur when our glucose and insulin levels are low.

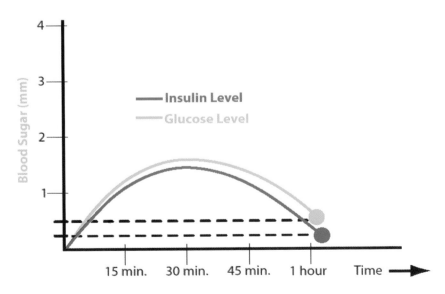

Oral Administration-Low Glycemic Carbohydrate

The Midriff Dragon Attacks the Liver

Insulin produces two major effects in the liver, which is one of the key organs involved in the regulation of our blood sugar. First, it slightly increases the rate of the metabolism of glucose. That is, it oxidizes glucose, or extracts energy out of the glucose molecule. It is this energy that our body uses for the many metabolic processes of all cells.

The second function of insulin in the liver is to use that energy in order to convert the rest of the glucose into a "storage form" of the energy molecule. This "storage form" is called **glycogen** and is simply a bunch of glucose molecules strung together in a long chain. Glycogen is like a fuel reserve tank in the liver that can be used when the body needs energy quickly. After a typical meal the body can store energy in this form, which can last us about eight hours.

If we do not replenish the glycogen stored in our liver through carbohydrate intake, then even if we are completely sedentary within twelve to twenty-four hours it will be completely depleted. However, if we are involved in strenuous and consistent exercise we may deplete this fuel stored in the liver within as little as 40 minutes.

In a healthy individual, if the sugar level in the blood decreases, so does the insulin level, and this causes the liver to then release the glycogen (stored fuel) to refuel the body during the fast between meals or if we need a quick burst of energy in a football game or an afternoon jog. The liver is like the gas tank in our cars that stores the fuel for the motor.

However, if there is an abundance of insulin in the blood, then the liver refrains from releasing the stored sugar (glycogen) because it assumes that the high presence of insulin means that there is plenty of sugar in the blood. In a normal person this feedback system insures that we safeguard our stored fuels for a time, in case our blood does not have the amount of glucose necessary to allow the many metabolic processes necessary for life to function. These stored glycogen molecules in the liver are then only released when our insulin level in the blood is low, signaling that our blood glucose level has depleted and we need fuel. Our body responds with hunger pangs that tell us it is time to go to the gas pump and refuel.

Unfortunately, this vital feedback system is compromised or short-circuited in obese or overweight people with midriff fat. Those of us who are battling the Midriff Dragon have a serious problem. The Midriff Dragon leaks fat into the liver from the visceral or midriff area, which alters the way the liver responds. The Midriff Dragon attacks the liver by leaking fat into it and keeping it from functioning as it is designed to do.

In other words, if there is fat in the liver (leakage from visceral fat), it alters the liver's response to insulin. It becomes resistant to insulin. This means that it will not sense the insulin. Subsequently the liver is deceived and releases sugar into the bloodstream unnecessarily, thinking that the blood is low on fuel. This causes the blood to have more sugar than it is supposed to have. At this point our gas tank is releasing too much fuel and it is flooding the carburetor. Adding to that problem, a liver with too much fat will also make more cholesterol and will therefore elevate the cholesterol level in the blood, which also contributes to cardiovascular disease.

This attack from the Midriff Dragon can therefore cause serious damage to our liver and reduce its ability to operate properly. Other functions that are imperative for the body to remain healthy are also fueled by glucose and are likewise facilitated by insulin (the key that opens the special channels). For example, the Kupffer cells in the liver use the energy of the glucose to detoxify our blood. This process is therefore of utmost importance in maintaining a healthy body. For this reason, a healthy liver is indispensable for us to remain in optimum health.

In addition, the glycogen stored in our livers is the primary fuel that energizes our brain. The brain is an extremely sensitive organ that requires a continuous and steady supply of blood sugar in order to function.   It is the most energy-demanding organ in our bodies and is responsible for over half the obligatory energy requirements of our system.

Except during starvation, the brain uses only carbohydrates (glucose) as a source of fuel. During starvation the brain can turn to ketones (produced from fatty acids) for energy but it is much less efficient in this regard.   In other words, the brain functions in an impaired state when not fueled by glucose. The muscles, on the other hand, can use both carbohydrates and fats as fuel with more efficiency. The glycogen provided by the liver is therefore essential for the brain to function optimally.

We can measure this dependence, for example, when we have prolonged levels of mental activity and our blood glucose levels drop. For this reason the consumption of carbohydrates is essential to cognitive processes, such as word recall, arithmetic, maze learning, short-term memory, rapid information processing, reasoning, and other measurements of intelligence.   Therefore, diets without any carbohydrates can have a significant reduction in these cognitive processes.

As we previously stated, if we have a diet which has no carbohydrates, within twelve to twenty four hours our glycogen stores in our liver will be depleted, even if we are totally sedentary. If we are involved in forty minutes of continuous intense physical exercises, we can completely deplete our glycogen stores within this short time. At this point, our body will begin to break down muscle protein to synthesize glucose for the brain and our nervous system to be able to operate. This, however, is insufficient and the brain then turns to the breakdown of fat so that it can make use of the ketones as an energy source.

When this happens, the level of ketones rises in our blood and gives us the fruity breath typically associated with this form of metabolism, but our mental capabilities are reduced in the process. The person feels sluggish, and since the glycogen stores in the muscle have also been depleted, even the idea of strenuous exercise of any kind becomes quite a challenge. People involved in such diets can scarcely motivate themselves to do any form of exercise.

The brain cannot tolerate excesses or deficits of sugar. It has a narrow parameter that must be strictly adhered to in order to function properly. That parameter is between 70 milligrams per deciliter (mg/dl) and 140 mg/dl.

Even if we fast the day before we take our blood sugar measurement, our blood sugar should not drop below 70 mg/dl. It is the liver's function to provide the timely release of this glycogen fuel in order to maintain the proper level of glucose in our blood that allows our brain to function within this tight parameter. A fasting blood sugar under 100 mg/dl is considered normal.

After a meal our blood glucose level rises, but normally this is no more than 140 mg/dl, and as the meal is digested it falls again. If a person has a fasting blood sugar of 126 mg/dl or greater, then he or she is considered to be a diabetic.

There are millions of people walking around today with pre-diabetic fasting blood sugar levels between 100 and 125 mg/dl. Alarmingly, they may not even know it because the symptoms have not yet become noticeable. These individuals are ticking time bombs ready to explode. Unless there are some changes in their diets they will inevitably cross the threshold into diabetes. It is only a matter of time.

If the blood sugar level drops below 60 mg/dl then the patient is considered to be dangerously hypoglycemic (low on sugar) and needs glucose to counter this deficit. Hypoglycemia (low blood sugar) is caused by unopposed insulin, or insulin without sugar in the blood. The brain will die without at least this minimum of glucose. This sometimes happens when a diabetic person takes insulin and then does not eat. Too much insulin in the body will cause one to go unconscious, because it completely depletes the glucose level in the blood and the brain shuts down. But mild hypoglycemia may also be a sign of impending type 2 diabetes, as we shall later see.

If the glucose level of the blood is either too high or too low for a prolonged period of time, it can also cause unconsciousness, serious brain damage, and even death. The importance of maintaining a healthy level of glucose and insulin in the body is therefore paramount in maintaining a healthy body. Either extreme can kill.

The elevated insulin level in the blood also affects the muscle tissue in similar ways. I t will stimulate the muscle to increase the utilization and the storage of the sugar in our blood. This allows us greater energy to use our muscles for physical activity. If we are not involved in activities, then the glucose is stored as fat. As a consequence, the more active we are, more of the blood sugar is burned and less is stored as fat.

We must therefore be leery of both extremes in diets. Diets without certain wholesome fats and proteins and which contain high glycemic carbohydrates are bad for our health. However, diets that have no low glycemic carbohydrates are also bad for our health. As we shall see, the right kind of carbohydrates consumed to fuel these metabolic processes will optimize our body's performance without harming other functions. In the final analysis, carbohydrates are necessary for proper brain function.

How High Glycemic Foods Trap Us with Our Midriff Dragon

The use of our second fuel tank enables us to reduce the size of our Midriff Dragon, but this process can only be activated if our insulin levels and our glucose blood levels are both low. The use of low glycemic carbohydrates will result in a low insulin spike and a low level of glucose in the blood. This allows the fat to convert to free fatty acids and depletes our fat stores. On the other hand, if the insulin levels are elevated, even when the glucose blood levels are low, the insulin will block the conversion of fats to FFA and therefore we will not metabolize our fat reserves.

Even though our first tank is low on glucose and the body is asking for fuel, the insulin will not allow us to use the second tank. It is as though a clamp has been placed on the fuel line leading to the motor from the second fuel tank.

4.1 - High insulin levels in the blood block the conversion of fat into free fatty acids that can be used for energy.

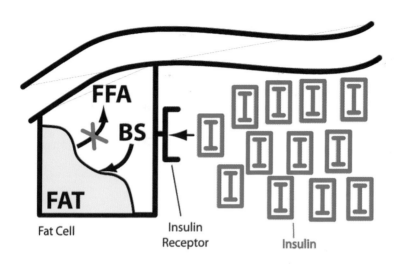

Fat Cell

Insulin Receptor

Insulin

This situation happens when we ingest high glycemic carbohydrates, which causes a rapid and high elevation of both insulin and blood sugar. Remember that insulin is the key that opens the special channels that allows the blood sugar to enter the cells for metabolism.

4.2 - High levels of insulin in our blood shut down the use of the second tank, even if the first tank is low on fuel.

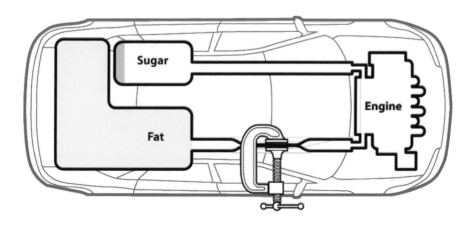

4.3 - *The ingestion of high glycemic carbohydrates causes a spike in insulin. The glucose is soon metabolized, but the insulin remains high for a period of time, blocking the use of the second fuel tank.*

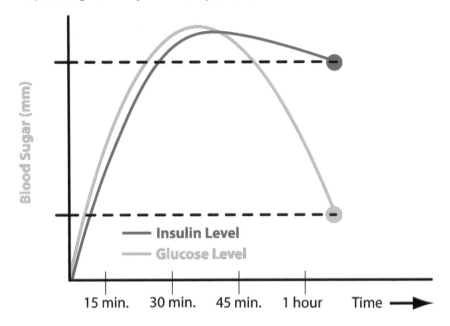

This high elevation of insulin causes an immediate and widespread opening of these special channels, resulting in a rapid drop in blood sugar levels. However, the insulin, being a large molecule that is much more difficult to eliminate, remains elevated and thus declines slowly. Because our level of blood sugar is low, the body would like to turn to the second fuel tank for its fuel needs, but because the insulin level remains high the conversion of fat to FFA is blocked.

The glucose level in our blood drops as it is used up in the cells. The insulin eventually drops also, although at a much slower rate. Once the insulin level is low enough in the blood, the body will automatically begin to use the stored fat as fuel. This is why the Atkins Diet works. It limits the intake of carbohydrates, forcing the body to resort to the stored fat as fuel.

But, it is also the reason why it won't work if you cheat. By eating high glycemic foods, the insulin spikes and stops the use of the second tank. However, we must understand that the quick and immediate weight loss in the first week is due also to the loss of the weight associated with our glycogen stores in the liver.

Anyone who has tried this diet knows that there is an immediate loss of about five to seven pd. in the very first week. This initial drop is the loss of the glycogen store in our liver that is burned off because no new glucose is being ingested. The loss of the stored glycogen and the four pd. of water associated with it often give people the impression that this rate can be maintained. It cannot. The loss in the following weeks is the true rate of fat loss in that diet.

This initial weight loss is quickly restored if one goes off the diet, with an immediate five to seven pd. gain. It is the weight lost in the following weeks that is the real accomplishment for the dieter, when the visceral fat is being burned as fuel. During this period, the person may feel sluggish and weak and their cognitive levels may suffer a little, as the brain is not at its best when fueled by ketones rather than glucose.

Moreover, if those following these diets cheat even a little and continue to ingest foods with a high glycemic index, then the body will immediately switch to the glycogen that will be produced in the liver, as the insulin levels in the blood rise, and then the body cannot resort to the stored fat as fuel, thus short-circuiting the whole idea. In this case, the foods with high protein content and the fat that are consumed as part of the diet will then not be metabolized but will instead be stored as more fat. The dieter will gain weight, rather than lose weight.

A Better Alternative

If we choose to eat carbohydrates with a low glycemic index, the insulin level in our blood will remain low and the body then preferentially chooses to leave this small amount of glucose alone to fuel the brain, which cannot easily use the energy from fat to function.

The strength of the Atkins Diet is that a person may lose visceral fat much quicker than in other diets, but its weakness is that most people cannot maintain this diet indefinitely. Strenuous exercise requires both fat and carbohydrate in the fuel mix. Therefore, few people can maintain an exercise routine of any great demand without ingesting some carbohydrates.

Those who are excessively overweight may choose this as a way to kick-start their diet with some substantial results, but in the long haul, if they do not moderate it slightly most people will not last. Furthermore, the diet may discourage the person from exercising, which is one of the foundational elements required to be a healthy person.

In addition, the Atkins Diet has two further drawbacks. The scarcity of carbohydrates leaves the dieter deficient in the proper amount of fiber, which is essential for a healthy colon. As a result, most individuals who follow this diet experience problems with constipation. Furthermore, this diet also leaves people deficient in the phytonutrients that are necessary for optimum health.

Hence, we would recommend a more balanced and scientific approach to adopting an eating lifestyle that allows you to prevent diabetes and lose the stored fats, while yet ingesting the right types of carbohydrates. Such an eating plan provides the necessary fiber and phytonutrients, which are indispensable for achieving and maintaining optimum health, while avoiding the negative aspects of a diet without any carbohydrates.

It is simply unrealistic to stay away from carbohydrates altogether for any prolonged period of time. Our intellectual performance requires carbohydrates. The brain is the most energy-demanding organ in our bodies, requiring almost half of the energy in our basic metabolic rate (BMR), our minimal obligatory energy requirement to stay alive. Other cells are not so restricted; most cells can use the fatty acids (glycerin) as a source of fuel. Thus, when we choose foods with a low glycemic index we provide some glycogen for our brain to use, and this also allows our body to automatically use the stored fats for fuel in other areas of our metabolism.

The best and most effective diet that can be maintained faithfully is one that includes low glycemic carbohydrates, a proper amount of the right fats, and a proper amount of proteins, making sure that the fiber content and the essential micronutrients necessary for optimum health are also included.

It is imperative that our choice of diet be one that we can maintain for the long run. Diets that cannot be permanently maintained are doomed to failure. If individuals revert to their previous habits, all benefits that were gained are soon lost. This leads to a vicious cycle that brings us despair.

The person who is serious about maintaining the right weight must understand that this requires a lifelong commitment and not a temporary fad. This commitment must include an exercise regimen that is realistic for the individual and which must be consistently applied. There are no quick fixes. Anything else is simply spitting into the wind.

Having fiber in our diets is essential to colon health and helps to produce satiety, the full feeling, which keeps us from overconsumption. The problem is that most refined foods and convenience foods, or fast foods, have very little fiber content and conceal fat, which overdoses us in calories before we feel full. These considerations together must not exceed the caloric output from ones' physical activity, through our daily routine and our exercise.

Moreover, if our diet avoids the high glycemic carbohydrates, we will avoid the insulin spikes and reduce the mechanism in our body that stores fats. We must keep in mind that high glycemic index carbohydrates are absorbed quickly in the gastrointestinal tract and will dramatically raise the blood sugar levels in our bloodstream, which will in turn result in an insulin spike and the storage of more fat that is deleterious to our health.

Conversely, low glycemic index carbohydrates are absorbed slower through the gastrointestinal tract. They do not raise blood sugar levels appreciably, and therefore they maintain low insulin levels that do not harm the body. As stated previously, insulin is a hormone that regulates the use of glucose (sugar) in our bodies. The human body is a marvelously engineered metabolic system that contains many complex feedback mechanisms. These feedback mechanisms attempt to maintain a careful metabolic balance (homeostasis) in order to efficiently provide us with the necessary functions that allow us to live. Without these feedback systems, we would not be able to convert foods into energy for the many functions that a living organism must have.

The relationship between glucose and the insulin hormone is an example of such a feedback system. Foods containing a high glycemic index, which can easily and rapidly elevate the blood-glucose level, will cause the body to secrete insulin accordingly. As we digest and absorb these high glycemic index foods, the glucose levels in our blood become proportionately elevated. In other words the intensity of the level of insulin in our blood is directly related to the level of glucose. If our levels of glucose are spiked by ingesting high glycemic meals, then our insulin levels will also be spiked high, in response to this rapid rise in glucose.

The Science

The Cause of Diabetes

After we ingest our meals, our digestive enzymes break down the molecules into smaller molecules that can be absorbed by our body. The glucose contained in that meal is absorbed in the gastrointestinal tract and then travels through our blood, reaching the pancreas.

Most of the cells in the pancreas are involved in the production and secretion of digestive enzymes. Here, specialized cells called beta cells and alpha cells in the Islet of Langerhans, are affected in two ways by the glucose. These specialized cells regulate the level of insulin in our blood. The beta islet cells produce a hormone called pro-insulin, while the alpha islet cells produce a hormone called glucagon.

An elevated level of sugar (glucose) in the blood stimulates the beta islet cells to produce proinsulin; meanwhile, the same high level of glucose in the blood causes the adjacent alpha islet cells to inhibit the production of another hormone called glucagon. The hormone glucagon acts antagonistically to insulin. In other words, they contradict one another. Thus, inhibiting the alpha cells from producing glucagon allows the proinsulin released by the beta islet cells to function freely without its restraining influence.

In short, the sugar in our blood turns on the production of proinsulin by the beta cells and stops the alpha cells from producing the hormone glucagon that would inhibit insulin.

5.1 - The production of insulin by the elevation of glucose in the blood.

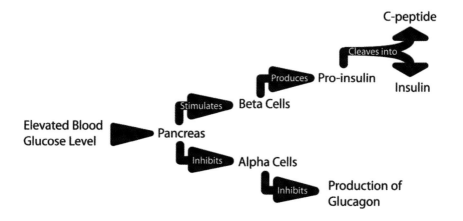

Imagine that two rival fraternities have their football players locked inside a room and being kept from the game behind their respective doors. The Proinsulin Fraternity is being kept behind the "beta" door, while the Glucagon Fraternity is housed behind the "alpha" door. This alpha door has an advantage in that if there is no one outside in the hallway the alpha door opens automatically, allowing the Glucagon team to exit the door and join in the game.

But the Proinsulin Fraternity behind the beta door has a plan. They have made a pact with another group to come and help them. This group, named Glucose, has arranged to send their members through the hall in order to foil the plans of the Glucagon Fraternity behind the alpha door. The Glucose group files past the alpha door and keeps pushing it closed so that the Glucagon group cannot get out. Also, as they go by the beta door they open it and allow the Proinsulin Fraternity to escape their room. The more Glucose members go through that hallway, the more Proinsulin members are freed to leave the room, while the alpha door remains shut.

The pro-insulin molecule, secreted by the beta islet cells, then cleaves, or separates into two separate molecules, insulin and C-peptide. In other words, the escaping Proinsulin fraternity splits into two teams, offense and defense. Where there is insulin in the blood we can find C-peptide, because they come from the same precursor molecule (proinsulin). This is useful to us in determining if a person is a type 1 or a type 2 diabetic.

While type 1 diabetics are not capable of producing the molecules of insulin and C-peptide, because their autoimmune systems have killed off the beta cells that produce it, the type 2 diabetic usually has some function of the beta cells. These have been damaged severely but not by the autoimmune system. There are other ways that we can damage these important cells. However, the type 1 diabetics cannot readily produce C-peptide because their beta cells have been destroyed by the autoimmune system. If we find a certain level of C-peptide in the blood, then it is a safe indicator that we are dealing with a type-2 diabetic.

You might ask, "What is an autoimmune system? How does it cause type 1 diabetes?" Normally our autoimmune system is what protects us from bacteria, viruses and any other pathogens that invade our bodies. Our autoimmune system is like the Coast Guard in the United States that protects our borders from invaders. If the Coast Guard would, instead of attacking our enemies, go haywire and begin to shoot down our own citizens peacefully fishing in their pleasure boats, it would become a problem for the welfare of our nation.

In much the same way, when the autoimmune system in our bodies incorrectly attacks certain cells within our organs, it becomes problematic. This is what happens in type 1 diabetes, as our autoimmune system destroys the beta cells, rendering them incapable of producing the molecule proinsulin that is normally converted to both insulin and C-peptide. This is the culprit that results in type 1 diabetes.

Type 2 diabetics, in contrast, usually have some insulin production capabilities although in diminished form. In this case, the beta cells are damaged by a different mechanism. When the glucose blood level remains high for a prolonged period of time, the beta cells are forced to work overtime. This prolonged activation of the beta cells damages them and causes them to go into shock, so that they can no longer produce the proinsulin molecule efficiently.

The beta cells begin to lose their ability to function and our body starts to lose its ability to create insulin. The result is that our blood glucose begins to rise, since there is no insulin to metabolize it. By testing for C-peptide we can therefore determine if the person has beta cells that are functioning at all, even if in a diminished state. If there is C-peptide present in the blood, then quite likely the patient is a type 2 diabetic.

5.2 - Insulin Receptors and Special Channels for Glucose

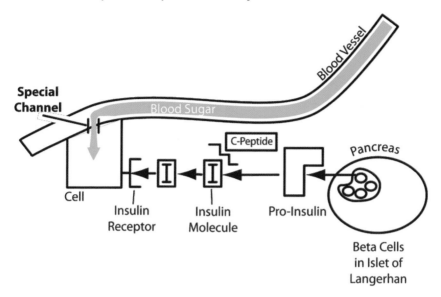

This insulin flowing through our blood now travels to a variety of organs and affects a wide number of cells in different ways. As it reaches the cells, it binds to special insulin receptors. These then serve as a key to open a "special channel" that allows the glucose or blood sugar to enter into the cell, so that it can provide the energy for whatever function the cell is designed to accomplish.

Without insulin, the cells have no way to open the special channels in the cells that allow the fuel (glucose) that is necessary to enter into the cell. Insulin is the key to the door. It is like the key to the gas cap in your car; without it you can't fill your tank, and eventually your car will stop running without fuel. Therefore, when there is no insulin in the body, the cells are starved for fuel.

Type 1 diabetics, who have little or no insulin in the body, will therefore usually be very thin and weak, as they are literally running out of fuel in their bodies. For our illustration to be more correct, the key would control a valve that allows the fuel from the tank to reach the motor. The tank may be full, but if the valve is not turned on there is no fuel reaching the motor and the engine stops running.

The glucose in type 1 diabetics remains in their blood and is not absorbed by the cells, so they cannot do the many metabolic processes required of life. The body attempts to rid itself of this excess sugar through frequent urination, which subsequently causes dehydration. This causes diabetics to have an unquenchable thirst. Their bodies even begin to draw water out of the surrounding tissues to further dilute the excess sugar in the blood, thus exacerbating the dehydration process even further.

Since they are not getting the caloric energy they need to metabolize through the transfer of glucose into the cells, the body begins to metabolize the stored fat for calories. For this reason type 1 diabetics are typically very thin, since all of their fat has been metabolized.

In the meantime, as the fat is being metabolized the type 1 diabetics are producing ketones as a byproduct, giving their breath a fruity smell. Ketones are acidic and their blood now begins to become too acidic, despite the body's attempt to blow out the acids through deep respirations.

If a type 1 diabetic does not have the right amount of insulin injected, or is dehydrated, the excess ketones in the blood then causes them to go into diabetic ketoacidosis (DKA), which will lead to coma and is potentially lethal. When the stored fat runs out, the body then begins to metabolize even the muscle and the organs, eventually causing death.

The Role of Obesity and Insulin in Type 2 Diabetes

In a normal person, with a normal level of blood glucose, as the insulin opens the "special channels" in the cells, the blood glucose enters into the cells and they are used as fuel. This process effectively uses up the glucose in the blood, and when the level subsequently drops, eventually the beta cells are given a break. The production of insulin stops, thus giving the cells the rest necessary to recuperate.

In other words, the subsequent lower blood glucose levels in the blood vessels, as glucose is being used in the cells, removes the stimulus in the beta cells to produce insulin. We have already discussed that the insulin level in the blood does not drop as quickly as the glucose level does. Because the insulin molecule is large, it takes much longer for it to be eliminated from the body. Therefore, even when the blood glucose level drops, the insulin level does not drop at the same rate.

The insulin level rises almost step-by-step with the rise in blood glucose, but it does not drop step-by-step with the glucose levels in the blood. If we are to give the beta cells a much needed coffee break, then we must avoid spiking the insulin too high so that it can be eliminated from the body before the next time glucose is ingested.

6.1 - Comparison of the drop of insulin in response to the drop in the level of blood glucose.

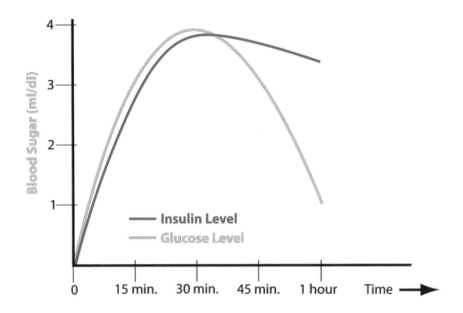

As you can see from the previous diagram, the level of insulin, once spiked by the ingestion of high glycemic foods, does not drop with the same speed that blood glucose does. It is for this reason that we do not want to create those high spikes in insulin levels. Once we spike the level too high, it takes a longer time to use up (metabolize) the insulin. This means that our blood insulin level remains continuously rather high in our blood.

When we keep insulin too long in our blood, it produces another problem. Not only are our poor beta cells being mercilessly whipped into a fevered pitch to produce the insulin when there is a continuous ingestion of glucose, but if the level of insulin is too high, even when ingestion is not as often, it keeps the beta cells working overtime.

When the level of insulin remains high in our blood, it now begins to overwhelm the receptor cells. Remember that the receptor cells are the keys that open the special channels to allow the glucose to enter into the cells. When insulin remains in our blood too long, the receptor cells are also being continuously assaulted, without an opportunity for a coffee break.

6.2 - The vicious circle of obesity, insulin resistance and type 2 diabetes.

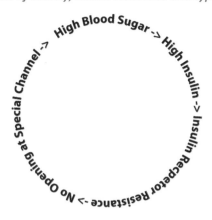

This continuous elevation of insulin in the blood causes the insulin receptors to become overwhelmed, as well. In response to this overstimulation, the receptors begin to become resistant to the insulin. This is called, "down regulation."

When the receptors "down-regulate" they no longer respond normally to the insulin, and they do not open the "special channels" that allow the blood glucose to enter into the cells. By disrupting the opening of these "special channels" the blood glucose cannot reach the cells and therefore remains in the blood, creating elevated blood glucose levels in the blood.

6.3 - The high levels of insulin cause the receptors to down regulate and keep the special channels closed. This does not allow the sugar in the blood to reach the cell and elevates the level of sugar in the blood.

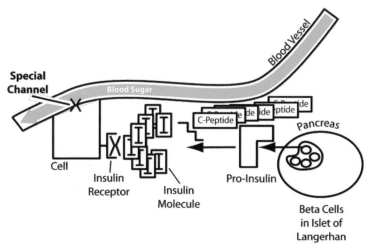

This adds insult to injury. Our poor beta cells in the pancreas are already being whipped to create more insulin by the high amount of glucose we are ingesting, but now the glucose in the blood is not being used up because the receptor cells are not opening the special channels. If the glucose cannot enter into the cells to be used as fuel, then it stays in the blood.

The increase in the level of glucose in the blood tells the beta cells that they need to produce even more insulin. The first taskmaster (high ingestion of glucose) had already whipped them into overdrive, but now a second whip (the increase in blood glucose due to the failure of the receptor cells to open the special channels) comes to spur them beyond their previous performance.

This begins a "catch 22" process. The poor beta cells being whipped by two taskmasters are now working double overtime and producing even more insulin. This elevates the blood insulin level even more, but in turn it further overwhelms the poor receptors, which are also being overworked, and they further down regulate in response to this increase in insulin.

The insulin receptor cells belong to a union, and they refuse to do more work, even when their assembly line increases in speed. Their response is to allow the assembly line to go past them untouched and they do even less work, allowing fewer glucose molecules to enter into the cells.

As these glucose molecules go by their assembly line untouched, they therefore remain in the blood and continue to elevate the glucose blood level. The industrious little beta cells are now watching all these glucose molecules going by and they go into emergency mode, working in 24-hour shifts to produce more insulin to cope with the excess glucose. Now they are not even sleeping at night. This vicious cycle continues until the poor beta cells have so many taskmasters whipping them that they finally become completely exhausted and can no longer work. At this point the person is a type 2 diabetic.

If the process is interrupted early enough to allow the beta cells to recover, there is a good chance that they can begin to function normally again. But if the wicked taskmasters continue to whip them for too long, they will quit altogether and resign from the job. In this case, the person is out of luck and must take insulin injections to artificially replace the work of the beta cells. They must outsource to another country (external source of insulin), but the work is never done as efficiently as before. Approximately one fifth of people with type 2 diabetes require insulin injections, just like type I diabetics.

This is why it is so important not to produce high spikes in our insulin production by ingesting high glycemic value foods. And it is the reason we should not be continuously ingesting glucose without giving the beta cells and the receptor cells a chance to rest. The lower we keep our insulin levels from spiking by ingesting foods with low glycemic index, the lower our daily insulin level will remain throughout the day. This reduces the enormous stresses on the poor beta cells and the insulin receptors, which would be continuously overwhelmed if the insulin levels remain high in our bloodstream.

Those type 2 diabetics fortunate enough, whose beta cells are still somewhat functioning, may be treated in one or more ways, either with medications that increase insulin secretion or medications that increase insulin sensitivity. But if the patient's beta cells have been too exhausted, they will need to take insulin injections.

The link between the over ingestion of high glycemic foods and the irreparable damage to the beta cells and the receptor cells is indisputable, and for this reason high glycemic foods should be avoided. However, the link between type 2 diabetes and obesity is equally as dangerous.

Lipotoxicity and Syndrome X

We have learned that insulin is the key that opens the special channels in our cells that allow the glucose to enter and provide the fuel it needs to function. We have also learned that high glycemic foods cause a spike in the insulin levels in our bodies, and if we do not give our beta and receptor cells rest we shall suffer the consequences of diabetes.

But, aside from continuous ingestion and high insulin spikes, there is another mechanism that causes insulin resistance. We have also learned that this high insulin level causes our body to store excess fat in our "second reserve tank." This excess fat overflows and leaks into the liver and interferes with its ability to sense insulin. In other words, it causes the liver to become insulin resistant.

This means that even when insulin is present, the liver does not sense it. Therefore, the liver thinks the blood glucose is low and subsequently releases glycogen (sugar) into the blood, further increasing the glucose level. This increase in glucose in the blood now forces the beta cells in the pancreas to produce more insulin in order to cope with the excess glucose. The poor beta cells are being whipped to work overtime, again with no coffee breaks. They cannot maintain that pace indefinitely. If they are not given a rest, they will burn out completely.

The overabundance of fat or adipose tissue also causes a syndrome we call "lipotoxicity." Lipotoxicity is created by high levels of circulating free fatty acids (FFAs) in the bloodstream, which have a direct toxic effect on the beta cells of the pancreas. It causes beta cell dysfunction, apoptosis, and diabetes. Furthermore, fatty acid overload in skeletal muscles causes insulin resistance, and in the myocardium (heart muscle) it impairs the cardiac function.

7.1 - Lipotoxicity is created by a spillover of free fatty acids to the blood.

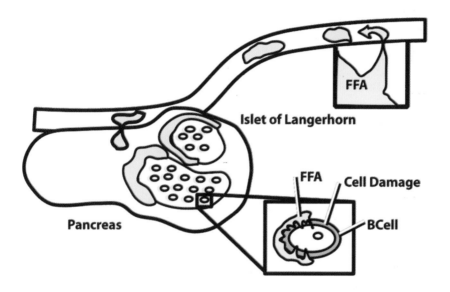

Lipotoxicity refers to the tissue disease that may occur when FFAs spillover in excess of the oxidative needs (the use of fuel) of those tissues due to over nutrition. In other words, when we have excess visceral fat (Midriff Dragon), it spills over and disrupts the normal functioning of the beta cells and the receptor cells. It causes them to also become insulin resistant.

This excess amount of FFAs enhances harmful metabolic pathways, which has toxic consequences. The amount of toxicity is directly dependent on the magnitude and duration of the imbalance in the overload. Overconsumption is therefore also a critical factor in the development of type 2 diabetes and in metabolic syndrome, which is sometimes referred to as "Syndrome X."

Approximately one third of obese adults, and perhaps as many teenagers, have Syndrome X, or insulin resistance syndrome. Over 60 million Americans have insulin resistance. Out of these, one in four will go on to develop type 2 diabetes.

This Syndrome X is a cluster of high-risk factors for diabetes and cardiovascular disease, such as high blood sugar, the Midriff Dragon (mid-girth more than 35 inches in women and more than 40 inches in men), high blood pressure, high levels of triglycerides and low density lipoproteins/LDL (bad cholesterol), and low levels of the good high density lipoproteins/HDL (good cholesterol).

As our metabolic processes come under attack by the high levels of insulin and the resulting obesity, we are given a lethal "three punch" combination that knocks us out of the ring. The result of these three punches leaves us with the deadly cluster of high-risk factors, which we call Syndrome X.

The First Punch: Insulin Resistance at the Receptor Level

We have learned that ingesting high glycemic carbohydrates elevates insulin levels that cause insulin resistance at the receptor level, which eventually leads to diabetes. This is the first punch, a hard jab to the chin.

The Second Punch: Lipotoxicity at the Cellular Level

We have also learned that this elevation of insulin causes obesity. This process begins a circular feedback loop that not only exacerbates the problem but also escalates it with time.

The obese individual now releases high levels of free fatty acids that deposit on organs such as the liver, beta cells, etc. These FFA deposits then have a direct toxic effect on the organ itself. The exhausted and overstimulated beta cells are now also being poisoned by the FFA, causing them further damage, so that the effect is now also in the cellular level as well as in the previous receptor level. Not only is the taskmaster whipping them harder, but now the factory they are working in is being attacked by terrorists who are spreading poisons to kill the workers. This is lipotoxicity. It is the second punch, a mean right cross that weakens our knees and makes us wobble on our feet.

7.2 - The vicious circle of obesity, lipotoxicity, and diabetes.

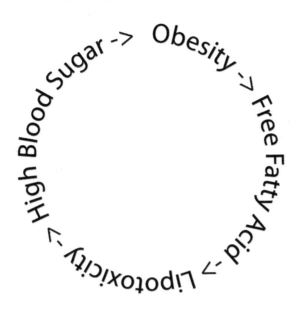

The Third Punch: Inflammation

It is of the utmost importance that we realize that Syndrome X can be attributed in large part to consequences brought about through visceral fat, or the Midriff Dragon. It is the Midriff Dragon that becomes the key component in the process that sends chemical signals that cause systemic inflammation.

We are all familiar with the inflammation of our sinuses when we have a cold. The cold virus triggers responses from our immune system to combat the particular pathogen. That induces the familiar inflammation, which causes our sinuses to become blocked and subsequently provides us with that misery common to the cold. But most of us are unaware that the overabundance of fat also triggers the chemical signals that lead to chronic inflammation throughout our bodies, and this includes our blood vessels. This inflammation turns out to be a critical aspect in many injurious processes, and it is precipitated by a cascade of responses from the immune system.

This systemic inflammation plays a significant part in cardiovascular disease. The inflamed blood vessels become constricted, and if there are cholesterol deposits on the walls the vessels will become contorted and may rupture pieces of the plaque. It can also cause small blood clots, which can produce equal damage. These may block the flow of a blood vessel to the heart, causing a myocardial infarction (damage to the heart muscle), or they may block a vessel in the brain, causing a stroke. This is the left hook to the chin, which knocks us out of the ring! It is the punch that knocks us into the Syndrome X and subsequently brings untold suffering and death to the unfortunates that become its victims.

The importance of the omega 3 and omega 9 fats, which come from monounsaturated and polyunsaturated oils like olive oil, cannot be underestimated, for they play a significant role in reducing this inflammation. Today we can identify people at elevated risks for heart attacks and strokes by testing blood for an inflammation marker called C-reactive protein (CRP). But the most effective way to stop this risk is to stop the Midriff Dragon from precipitating all the elements that comprise syndrome X to begin with.

This means that we must stop overconsumption, exercise adequately, and eat the right kinds of foods, those that do not exacerbate the storage of visceral fats. We must defeat the Midriff Dragon if we are to defeat diabetes and the many disastrous medical complications it produces. There are no short cuts.

Heart attacks and strokes kill about three-quarters of people with diabetes. In other words, if you have diabetes you have a 75% chance of dying by either a heart attack or a stroke. This means that if you have diabetes your chances of dying from a heart attack are just as high as the risk faced by someone without diabetes who has already had a heart attack.

For some reason, this risk is greater for women than for men. According to the 2004 report in Archives of Internal Medicine, women who have diabetes have a 150% increased risk of a heart attack, while men have an increase of 50%.

Hypoglycemia - A Warning

Hypoglycemia is usually a warning of future problems with diabetes. It is caused by having too much insulin and too little sugar in the blood. It can happen to type I diabetics who take an insulin shot and do not eat afterwards. The lack of glucose in the blood causes hypoglycemia. But this may also happen to people who are not diabetics yet. By ingesting high glycemic foods, which spike our insulin, we can also experience hypoglycemic episodes.

In order to illustrate the difference between the effects of low glycemic diets and high glycemic diets in the course of a day, we shall use two fictional characters and study the effect of their different diets through the course of a day. Our first character is High Glycemic Henry. Henry starts his morning at 7:00 AM with a high glycemic breakfast of doughnuts, waffles, and a healthy portion of syrup. His blood glucose elevates rapidly, and this triggers a subsequent and explosive response in the level of insulin in his blood.

In Fig. 10.1, the red line represents Henry's level of insulin and the green line represents his level of blood sugar. As a result of High Glycemic Henry's high insulin levels, by mid morning his blood sugar levels have bottomed out. The sugar is quickly metabolized and then the levels plummet. However, because of the high insulin level he cannot access the second fuel tank and is prevented from using the fat stores as an alternate fuel source. At 9:30 in the morning his unopposed level of insulin is causing him to become hypoglycemic.

8.1 - High GI Henry's seesaw

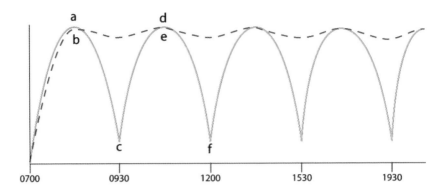

The low blood sugar precipitates a cascade of responses. Henry is now becoming very irritated and has developed the jitters and shakes. His heart rate is also elevated. His body is telling him that he needs to correct this problem. Therefore, Henry now has tremendous hunger pangs. Henry is driven by his hunger pangs to consume another high glycemic index meal that will satisfy his urge. This will cause another rapid rise in his blood sugar, which provides for him a temporary relief from his symptoms but once again sends his insulin levels sky high. Again, because of this high insulin level, his blood sugar will drop like a rock as the insulin quickly dispatches the glucose into the cells.

By lunchtime our unfortunate friend is once again in the same predicament he was in during mid morning. He is irritable and has the shakes. His hunger pangs return in full force because he cannot access the alternate fuel source, which is being blocked by the high insulin level. Once again, Henry consumes another high glycemic index meal to relieve his ravenous hunger. As you can observe in the Fig. 10.1, this seesaw continues throughout the entire day.

In the end, Henry's insulin levels have remained elevated all day long. This predisposes Henry to the many problems mentioned earlier. The high level of insulin creates the previously discussed down regulation of the receptors, which leads to type 2 diabetes. It not only keeps him from using the stored fat, but it also causes a greater storage of fat, resulting in obesity. These are the contributing factors that lead to diabetes and Syndrome X. It should be noted that diabetes in turn is the precursor to an enormous number of other illnesses that ravage our bodies.

Our second character in this daily drama is Low Glycemic Linda. Linda begins her morning with a breakfast of low glycemic fruits and a protein shake. She avoids the typical morning processed cereals that are generally of a high glycemic value. In this respect our European brothers have a much healthier alternative to the typical American breakfast. They usually have some form of meat or other protein with wholegrain bread. Linda's low glycemic meal creates a slow rise in blood sugar, which concurrently causes a slow rise in her insulin.

The low level of insulin in Linda's blood has subsequently maintained a stable blood sugar level throughout the day. Additionally, the low level of insulin allows her to access the second fuel tank. Linda is therefore reducing the fat stores in her body. She is not experiencing the adverse symptoms that High Glycemic Henry suffered (jitters, shakes, and hunger pangs).

As you can see in Fig. 10.2, Linda has had ample fuel for her needs throughout the day, using stored fats to supplement her blood sugar. Her low levels of insulin and blood sugar allow her to tap into the second tank for extra fuel. Not only has Linda reduced the amount of stored fats, but she has also avoided the high levels of insulin that bring on the cascade of illnesses associated with it.

Linda, unlike Henry, has the energy to work and exercise, while avoiding the tremendous hunger pangs created by insulin spikes. This not only allows her to be more mentally attentive but also gives her an even emotional state throughout the day. Moreover, when she is done with her work she will have the energy to exercise.

8.2 - Low GI Linda maintains a stable insulin to glucose level.

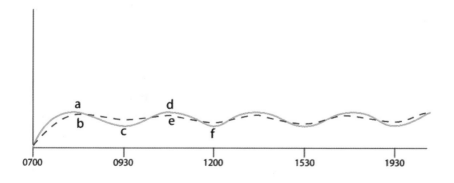

If we are to lead healthy and productive lives, we must become aware of the icebergs that lurk about us, waiting to sink our ship. We must learn to eat the right foods in moderate amounts and we must plan to exercise daily. Our modern sedentary lives are no longer physically demanding. Therefore, if we hope to live long and productive lives, we must take the time to exercise. Simple changes in our choices, like taking the stairs rather than the elevator, or walking rather than riding somewhere, can mean the difference between staying trim and gaining fat.

Low impact exercises like swimming or riding a bicycle are recommended for those who are suffering with joint problems and or are extremely overweight. The excess weight plays havoc on our joints. Those who do not correct their obesity are condemned to face serious joint problems as they get older. It may now seem trivial to some, but it will not be trivial when the pain in your hips and knees do not even let you sleep at night.

In addition to leading sedentary lives, people today are confronted by food that is not only more abundant than ever before but laced with sugar by modern marketing geniuses who have realized that in doing so it increases consumption. This clever tactic increases the glycemic value of much of the products we buy from our grocery stores. Sadly, this practice has been especially geared by the greedy merchants to target our children. The use of cartoons and many other Madison Fifth Avenue production tools have carefully seduced our children to buy their sugar-laced products. Many parents in this generation have become ignorant accomplices to this crime against our little ones.

Furthermore, many new industrial processes in food production have created other pressing problems. In the past, grains were stone ground and the flour created by this process was thicker and coarser than today. The larger grain provided less surface area for the enzymes to attach, and this slowed down the digestion and absorption process, subsequently lowering the glycemic index. Modern steel rollers used to ground grains create very fine flour, whose smaller size gives it greater surface area and allows it to be more easily reached by the digestive enzymes. This causes a more rapid absorption rate and an immediate spike in the blood-glucose level, which causes our body to produce an overabundance of insulin in response. For this reason, white bread has such a high glycemic value and all baked goods using white flour have similar results. It must be also noted that the cooking of carbohydrates causes them to soften and swell, again offering a greater surface area for the digestive enzymes to attach and to more rapidly digest it. The carbohydrates we ingest in many cafeteria-style restaurants, where food is cooked in mass quantities and then kept warm for long periods of time, are extremely overcooked and easily absorbed by the body, creating a higher glycemic value. For this reason, it is a good policy to always cook things al dente in order to lower the glycemic index.

Sadly, canning and precooking foods not only destroy many of the vitamins in the process but also cause the foods to have a higher glycemic index. It is a better choice to purchase fresh vegetables whenever possible. All of these modern trends in our eating habits translate into big problems for our health. For our bodies to function in our modern society at an optimum level we must be aware of the kinds of foods we ingest and the amount of fuel they will store in our system. Simply stated, if we store more energy than our bodies can effectively use, it will create an overabundance of fat that will negatively impact our health and work against our benefit.

In summary, we must understand that all foods that contain carbohydrates are eventually turned into glucose in our bodies. This sugar then stimulates the secretion of insulin, which allows us to use the glucose in our varied metabolic processes and to store the excess as fat. Not all carbohydrates are created equal. Some, with a high glycemic index, will produce a higher blood glucose level and will subsequently cause a person to store more fat. Moreover, if we continuously keep our blood sugar levels high, the fat we have stored will not be metabolized. As a result, the incidence of obesity has reached the pandemic level in our nation and is rapidly becoming the most serious medical and economic problem in the world.

Low-fat diets that do not incorporate the proper use of the glycemic index are therefore incomplete and ineffective in allowing the body to burn off the excess stored fat, which causes so many negative side affects to our health. For our exercise routine to be effective in tapping our second tank, we must keep our insulin and blood sugar levels to a minimum. If our insulin level is high, we will only burn the glycogen in our primary fuel tank (the liver). A minimum of 20 minutes of a sustained exercise, which brings your heart rate to 80% of its maximum capacity, is recommended in order to best accomplish this goal. Individuals with cardiac problems should consult their cardiologist to determine their personal parameters. Obviously, for non-cardiac patients, the more time you add to this exercise regime the better results you will get.

By burning off our visceral fat, all of us, regardless of our body mass index, can avoid the inflammation that leads to arteriosclerosis and heart disease. The use of the glycemic index should therefore not be limited to diabetics or morbidly obese people.

The use of the glycemic index in choosing the foods we ingest is absolutely essential and indispensable for everybody, every day, and every meal, if we are to enjoy the fruit of living in optimum health.

Hyperphagia and the Obesity Vortex

Earlier in the book, we mentioned that our modern culture has succumbed to three major stumbling blocks that have led us into the Age of Globesity. These stumbling blocks are:

1. **Because of our sedentary lifestyles, we are burning fewer calories.**
2. **We are eating the wrong types of foods, which are easily converted to fat.**
3. **We are eating more than ever.**

These three elements work synergistically to create the nation's rising trend in clinical obesity. And the epidemic is spreading around the globe, as nations join our culture in the consumption of fast foods and in our habit of overconsumption. We have crossed the threshold into the Age of Globesity.

Today, Americans spend nine times as many minutes watching television and movies as they do all other leisure activities combined. The computer age has brought our children out of the playgrounds and parked them in front of their video games and the computers.

Not only are the manufacturers creating foods that are high in glycemic index, but the retailers are supersizing our nation into the grave. The average caloric intake for an American male has increased by 168 Kcal/day in the last 30 years, and the average caloric intake for American women has increased by an astounding 335 Kcal/day in the last 30 years.

This, by itself, is extremely critical, but it is exponentially compd.ed by the high glycemic foods we now ignorantly consume. In other words, not only are we eating much more than we need to function correctly, but the foods we are eating are causing us to have an elevated insulin level that brings with them dire consequences.

These various elements conspire to bring our nation to its knees through the future burgeoning cost of medical care. We have explained how eating the wrong type of carbohydrates can lead us into diabetes and the many related pathologies. It is essential to understand that all three of these elements must be addressed if we are to gain control of this dire trend, which shall lead us into financial chaos.

We would like to supersize your health and draw your foot from the grave, placing the other one away from the banana peel and into the gym. We have given you the information you need to make the right choices that will lead you to a healthier and happier life, but it is up to you to make that choice.

Here is where the rubber meets the road. In the end, it is up to you to choose what path you will take. Some of you have difficulty in this area. There are psychological reasons for this problem. We cannot, therefore, complete our discussion without addressing the issue of hyperphagia (overconsumption) and the psychology behind it.

There are significant psychological factors involved in people who have problems with hyperphagia. It is important to understand that this cannot be lightly treated or ignored. But, the reader must understand that if there is to be any real headway in avoiding obesity and the many health pitfalls involved with it, then our caloric intake cannot be greater than our caloric output. This is essential.

There are, thus far, no magic pills. If we increase our consumption, we must increase our exercises accordingly or we end up storing fat. The problem is that there are a growing number of people that eat more than they could realistically burn. You can eat all the right foods and even exercise on a daily basis, and yet, if you eat more than you can possibly burn you will gain weight.

I had a patient once who came to me complaining that the glycemic index did nothing to help her lose weight. Betty was in her mid thirties and weighed over 300 lbs. Her weight gain had come mainly after she was married in her early twenties. She was now in her early forties. Sadly, her obesity eventually led to her divorce. My heart was broken for her sad situation, and I wanted desperately to help her.

After investigating the types of foods that she ate and the amounts ingested, I showed her that she was eating ten times the amount of food that a normal female of her height should be eating. Even if she kept only to low glycemic index foods, the total amount of calories she was ingesting simply could not be burned by her physical activity and was bound to end up as stored fat.

An average man with an average activity level should consume approximately 2,228 calories per day. An average woman should consume 1,782 calories per day. If you increase your physical activity to burn more calories than what you ingest, then the body must burn the fat in reserve to make up the difference. When this happens the person loses weight. On the other hand, if you ingest more than you burn, then the body stores the excess energy in fat. There is no magic to the system.

Betty was caught in the "obesity vortex," a spinning vortex that drags all who are caught within it deeper into hell. Every time she was depressed, Betty was conditioned to overcome her sadness by eating. Perhaps her unwary parents precipitated this when she was a baby. I have watched exasperated parents shove a bottle into their baby's mouth the moment they begin to cry.

A baby is not hungry every time he or she cries. As a matter of fact, the digestive system of a baby needs to have time to digest the previous meal. For babies as well as adults, eating between our meals interferes with the proper functioning of the digestive system. It is no wonder that these children become colicky.

By shoving a formula bottle into their babies' mouths every time they cry, parents begin to build a pattern that can cause great damage in the future, not realizing that their actions have far reaching consequences in the future health of their children.

Betty was depressed over her weight and found refuge in the refrigerator, but this only exacerbated her problem and drew her into the obesity vortex. Once her stomach was enlarged by gorging herself, it became very difficult for Betty to eat less. By continuing to overeat, her stomach continued to stretch and the vortex spun with ever increasing speed. The problem is that if Betty does not stop the vortex it will eventually kill her.

It has been my observation that hyperphagia is an addiction, no less seductive and no less powerful than cocaine or heroin addiction. But it is not a hopeless situation. It can be changed when a person really wants to change it. The number one rule in treating drug addicts is that nobody can help them until they really want to be helped. The same applies to people with food addiction.

The cause of the addiction must be confronted. It is not possible to overcome the problem only through attempts to correct the symptoms. If we do not address the underlying cause that produces the symptoms, we shall fail. It is no different than being addicted to any other substance; the psychological causes must be addressed. Furthermore, the individual must come to the point in his or her life that he or she truly wants to stop the addiction. Only when we come to the point that we admit our need for help can we begin the process of healing.

Some of us must hit the absolute rock bottom before we become truly convinced that we want to change. When people with an addiction problem come to me and say they can't help it, I always say, "No, that is incorrect. What you are really saying is, 'I don't want to change badly enough yet.' If you really wanted to change, you could." Of course, there are steps that must be taken; twelve-step programs have been shown to be quite productive in helping people with addictions.

It is time that we begin to view hyperphagia as an addiction. Too often, in our politically correct culture, we treat obesity at the same level as a paraplegic or some other handicapped group. Of course, I am not insinuating that we treat obese people with disrespect. All human beings have infinite worth and value, as created in the image of God, regardless of their sex, color, age, financial status, intelligence, abilities, physical appearance, weight, or any other superficial categorization we can make. The worth of an individual is not based on any physical properties of the individual. It is an intrinsic value that was recognized by the founding fathers of this great nation. For this reason they wrote that we were endowed by our Creator with certain unalienable rights.

But while the paraplegic cannot change his or her situation, the addict cannot claim the same excuse.

We do not view smokers as a minority group with special privileges. The habit is injurious to the health of the individual, and it can be changed. The same applies for obesity. The evil we are here confronting is not the person, but rather the addiction. If we begin to see the gravity of the consequences that obesity brings to our health, family and collective culture, then we can begin to address the problem. If we do so, then we will find that the very same principles that empower addicts to overcome substance abuse can empower those who are plagued with the need or psychological dependency for overconsumption.

There are some few cases where metabolic imbalances, such as thyroid insufficiencies, may cause obesity. These are not caused by psychological reasons, but must be treated medically. However, they do not compose the vast majority of cases, where obesity can be changed through behavioral modifications.

All human beings establish patterns during their lives. When repeated often enough, these patterns become habits and habits create behavior modifications. If we habitually eat when stressed, then we are leaving ourselves at the mercy of our environment and the stresses that we must face. These control us, rather than us controlling them.

Such behavioral problems can be changed, but they must first be confronted. Comfort foods provide many of us with the psychological influence to indulge beyond the limits of what is healthy. We sacrifice our long-term safety for a short-term comfort. We sell out our entire future health for the immediate gratification of our senses. It may feel good in the moment, but the devil is in the contract and the pleasure is never worth the suffering it will later produce.

The sex addict faces the same dilemma. The pleasure becomes the addict's god. This cannot be overcome until the consequences of this error becomes so negative that the individual is personally convinced that the pleasure is not worth the pain that it later produces. It is usually at this point that the addict can come to the door of healing. Only when the addict has become really convinced that this habit must change can the healing begin. No one can force that decision on anyone else. It must come from the individual.

There is yet another sector of our society that has great difficulty with overconsumption. Some people who have been raped or abused in any way end up having a problem with self-loathing. They feel that somehow they are unworthy and in their self-hatred they subconsciously do things to hurt their body. These individuals must seek professional help to overcome the underlying causes of their addictions. Their symptoms may be expressed in forms of addictions to sex, drugs, foods, or many other compulsive behavioral patterns.

If there is anything that we say that is worth hearing, it is this: You are not a zero. You have infinite worth and value as a human being created in the image of God, regardless of your weight. You are precious and unique in every way. Hear us when we tell you this: Who we are is not what has happened to us! We are whom we choose to be. Our worth is not determined by our outward appearance.

To be sure, our outward appearance does impact us in many ways. We are not denying this. The sad truth is that in a competitive market, employers will often choose to hire those who are not overweight from a purely financial point of view. They consider overweight persons to be greater liabilities, because statistics show that they will be more apt to miss work due to medical complications.

Nevertheless, our motivation for losing weight ought never to be governed by our acceptance from others. This is a trap that must be avoided. Our true and proper motivation should be to live a healthy and productive life. Our self-esteem should never be based on externals, but rather on the internals.

The Psychology of a Healthy Lifestyle

By Paul Rodriguez, M.D.

Kate and Alice had made a pact never to tell anyone, and now Alice is dead. During their teens, both girls had suffered from a disorder known as anorexia nervosa, but Alice had it worst. Their parents had been too busy, too involved to notice, and they had managed to keep it a secret, until it was too late.

That was years ago, and Kate switched over to bulimia a while back. But the pain and the guilt are still there, deep, intractable... and she treats them with all the comfort food she can get her hands on. Bingeing... feeling guilty and bloated... purging... feeling empty... bingeing again... Lately, Kate has taken to drinking; it helps her to make it through the night.

Adding fuel to this pernicious cycle is the realization that the slim, youthful Kate has been replaced by this overweight and washed out version of herself. The repeated metabolic insults have progressively ravaged her body. Dull, brittle hair, etched teeth that have lost most of their enamel, enlarged parotid glands that make her look like she has a permanent case of the mumps... She feels ugly, helpless and hopeless. And the secretive life she still lives has cut her off from that which she needs now more than ever: human love and acceptance.

Then there is Mark, who has been living with *Dunlap's disease*. At first he thought it was funny ("Look y'all, my belly's *dun lapped* over my belt!"). Cute. After his first heart attack Mark should've known better. Year after year, Mark had watched his belly grow and spill over his belt, until a belt didn't cut it and he had to start wearing suspenders.

When his family doctor began to nag him about it, Mark wasn't ready to hear it. He liked his food, chips, and beer too much to even think about making a change. Besides, his family, neighbors and friends were all overweight (some much more than he). No one else was trying to change their eating habits, so why should he?

It took a second heart attack that nearly bought him a ticket to the death experience, and landed him in the cardiac intensive care unit, to pull his head out of the sand. Now, Mark sees his son, Tom, and his daughter, Lydia, with different eyes: they both are already overweight and heading for certain obesity, rushing toward the devil's triangle of diabetes, hypertension, and cardiovascular disease. He knows what a terrible example he has been for his family and is feeling the guilt of it gnawing at him every day. Mark *wants* to change—but can he, after so many undisciplined decades of gluttony?

Now Mary's is a different story. Mary has no problem controlling her weight, but her obsession with control has become her merciless master. Image maintenance has been an overtime job with her. Slim, trim, able to wear anything and look good, she has not let her guard down in more years than she can count. Ruled by the mortifying fear of becoming fat (that unpardonable sin!), Mary is an accomplished inspector of every morsel that crosses her lips and an infallible detector of cellulite or unwanted millimeters on her waistline or hips. She has never learned to laugh at herself, and she will never allow herself to fail at anything. Anything. The envy of some of her less-than-perfect friends, she looks like the specimen of physical health. Yet Mary is not mentally, emotionally, or spiritually healthy at all; and a closer look tells us that her physical health has greatly suffered for this. Deep inside, she longs to be free.

We may read these stories and comfort ourselves with the thought that we are nothing like these poor, miserable, neurotic people. But on closer inspection some of us will find that our lives (or the life of someone near and dear to us) are variations of these themes. In fact, many of us may identify, to some degree or another, with Mark and his family. Some of us will catch painful glimpses of ourselves in the lives of Kate or Mary. Otherwise, why would we be reading this book? When it comes to the heart of the matter, we are usually the last ones to know, are we not? So, if we can cut through the fog of denial for a moment, let us look at what it takes for us to be free to live a healthy life—or, more accurately, to discover the healthy you.

Bookseller's shelves are filled with how-to books on dieting, weight loss, healthy eating and exercise. Television shows feature the experts reiterating their newest advice and strategies on these subjects. But, despite this unprecedented degree of exposure and wealth of information at our fingertips, more and more of us find ourselves on the deadly path that leads to obesity and its morbid complications. Why is that? Why do we continue to fail as individuals and a society in this key area of our lives?

First, let's take a look at plain and simple overeating. As in Mark's case, overeating boils down to a bad habit for most of us. It grows out of self-comforting behavior that has been reinforced over and over again (or, as the behaviorist would say, "over learned") since most of us were children.

We have been taught to find comfort in food. Mom, dad, grandma, grandpa (you name it) expressed their love for us through feel-good foods such like cookies, cake, and ice cream. For us, feasting on these foods became a central part of Christmas, Thanksgiving, weddings, etc., so we've associated these foods with special good feelings. Even for those of us who were abandoned, neglected, or abused, comfort foods had a positive impact in the way we felt: they served as consolation and contrast to the toxic, feel-bad lives we were forced to live. When we feel empty, sad, bored, hurt, angry... these foods are there to comfort us.

Purveyors of snack foods have long been aware of the power of this feel-good effect; it is the first step on the road to addiction, and they would definitely love for us to become addicted to their products. Like any other object of addiction (alcohol, drugs, sex, or pornography), comfort foods give us that emotional "fix" we crave. No need to psychoanalyze it. Given enough time, overeating will lead to addictive behavior. And if we want to be successful in overcoming it, we must meet it head on and treat it like an addiction. Nothing less.

There are many proven tools and methods available to treat addiction, but the key element to change is *commitment*. We also know that commitment is most effectively fueled by our internal motivation. It is essential then that we harness two very important motivational forces: what I call the *misery* (or cost) of our addictive behavior, and the *good life* (a life that is free from addiction and rewards us with the fruit of a healthy, fulfilling existence—the kind of life we were all meant to live).

Let us take on the misery first. Many of us are not motivated to change because we don't realize how miserable we truly are. None of us like to look at the messes we have created along the way, none of us want to look at the real cost of the bad decisions we all have made during the course of our lives. Like Mark before his second heart attack, most of us prefer to be like the ostrich, with its head buried in the sand, oblivious to the mess we have made, blissfully unaware of the terrible storm heading our way. This is denial. And denial keeps us walking blindly along the deadly path.

Yes, the truth often hurts and, of course, no one likes to feel the pain—so we run to do everything and anything we can to numb the pain and forget that it was ever there. But *pain is a great motivator*—it can become a friend that opens our eyes and keeps us from falling down the cliff of eventual self-destruction. Dr. Frank Patino wrote this book because he clearly saw where we (especially our children) are headed; he wrote it to open our eyes.

If we allow it, his book will serve to do for us what it was intended to do: to free us to live a healthy, fulfilling life. For this, we need the courage to open our eyes wide and count the cost of our behavior. We need to see where this behavior has led us in the present. And we need to look ahead to the dismal future our behavior is creating for us (and for our loved ones who follow our examples).

Now, let us look at the good life—the life of freedom from this addiction—that awaits us. *Without hope there is no sustainable change.* Being committed to escaping the misery and abandoning the road to destruction we find ourselves walking isn't enough. We all need to have a life, a purpose, to pursue.

But many of us were discouraged early on from knowing who we are, from finding our individual path in life, from wanting the kind of life that was meant for us. It may have been parents, teachers, or any other powerful significant person in our early lives, but the self-defeating messages were there, penetrating into our little souls and robbing us of the hope and courage we needed. *You will never make it. You will always be a failure. Don't even think about success, or you'll be let down every time. You can't trust anything that looks promising. You don't have a right to your dreams. Accept your life, the way it is now, and you won't get hurt....* Get the point? (Please remember that the point is not to blame anyone for this—blaming never frees us—the point is to understand.)

When we accepted those lies about ourselves as gospel truth, day after day, year after year, we allowed them to keep us from seeing the true possibilities of our lives. Defeat became a way of life. Feeling helpless and unfulfilled, we turned to anything that brought us comfort and helped us ease the pain.

Ironically, in doing this we sabotage our recovery and freedom—and we keep on adding to the walls others initially built for us, raising them higher and higher with each passing year. As long as we accept and believe the self-defeating messages issuing from our heads, from our memories—and as long as we try to fix the negative emotion such messages generate in us—we keep ourselves from catching a clear, unhindered vision of the life that is possible for us, of the life that is waiting for us out there.

Like so many of us out there, Robert had lived all his life under the shadows of his brilliant sister and his jock brother. When he wasn't ignored, he was compared to them by his father and always found wanting, falling short of the mark. Mother saw and wept in secret, and she took every opportunity to comfort her son when father wasn't looking. For Bobby, food became the most reliable currency of love. By the time he reached middle school, the tag "Tubby Bobby" had permanently stuck to him. He had become a ready target for the boys (the girls were too polite to say anything to his face—or, did they even care?). He had become the butt end of many a joke.

Bobby had always loved sports, but he had never dared to try out. He remembered how his father and brother had such a great time at his expense, roaring with laughter at the idea. How could Tub ever keep up with the others? Why, he probably wouldn't even make the first cut in the girls' team. At any rate, the thought of showering in the locker room, naked, in front of the other boys, gave Bobby the shivers. So he settled for watching sports on the tube and comforting himself with the company of his "reject" friends, chips, sodas, and as much of mother's baked goodies as he could get his hands on.

He tried dieting, but the shed pd. of fat would boomerang on him with a vengeance. And although his growing obesity served to insulate him from the relationships he craved, it also protected him from the pain of inevitable rejection. Bobby knew he was miserable, but loneliness was better than rejection.

Like the rest of us, Bobby once had dreams. When he was a kid, he remembered wanting to be like his Uncle Luke—the soldier, the family's war hero—more than anything else in the world. But it was a dream that ended up with all the others in the dark and dusty attic of his childhood memories. Until the day he saw the poster, and the resemblance to Uncle Luke jolted him out of complacency.

The marine was pointing at him, promising to shape him into the person he had secretly wanted—but was afraid—to be, promising the life he had always wanted. So, with the hope that comes with the resurrection of a dream, Robert found the courage to walk into the recruiting station and apply for enlistment.

Naturally, the marine recruiter took one look at him and shook his head, but Robert wasn't daunted. He asked the man how much weight he would have to lose and said he would be back. The recruiter patted Robert on the back, wishing the young man good luck, and shook his head again the moment Robert stepped out on the sidewalk.

Without a doubt, the negative, self-defeating messages kept replaying inside Robert's head for some time, but he had caught the vision and was committed to it. He gave up his sodas, beer, chips, and sweets. He gave up all starchy foods (foods with a high glycemic index), along with the excess of dairy products he had been accustomed to consuming.

He had found his true goal, his purpose, and a passion that began to swallow up every self-defeating message that stood in his way. Keeping his vision before him at all times, he filled the hunger with anything and everything that would help him get a step closer to his goal.

He began to lower his insulin resistance by walking, then speed walking, then jogging for longer periods of time. He joined the Y and started working out and swimming regularly. He stayed away from vending machines, and he began to spend less and less time in front of the boob tube and more time feeding his mind and strengthening his spirit. And the positive results he was experiencing encouraged him to keep on keeping on.

At first, his friends laughed at him (they winked at each other and told themselves it was just a phase that would soon blow over). With time, however, they started to believe Bobby was serious about this, too serious to be sidetracked by any flippant remark or note of skepticism coming from them. But Robert's father and brother were another story; their lack of faith in him still cut deep.

On the other hand, Robert had begun to collect a new set of committed friends whom he met at the Y and the track, like-minded who were impressed by his commitment and were ready to challenge him to renew that commitment whenever he dragged in, feeling sorry for himself and licking his wounds. With time, Robert learned to keep his eye on the goal and steel himself against the barbs of the unbelievers.

Mother worried about him (she always did). She said he was too "skinny" and offered him his favorite foods. But Robert simply smiled, hugged her and told her that her love was all he wanted. She cried and blinked back the tears, then stepped back to take a closer look and witness the metamorphosis that was gradually transforming her Bobby….Six months later, Robert walked into the marine recruiting station with the step and the look of a man who knows where he's going in life.

It's never too late to allow ourselves to dream the good dream, to envision and move on into the kind of life we will have as we become free from all that hinders us, slows us down, poisons us, and slowly destroys us. So what is it going to be then, another five, ten, even twenty years of believing the negative, self-defeating messages about our selves? Does it have to take another five, ten, or twenty years of mounting misery? Another five, ten, or twenty years of moving further and further away from the kind of life we've always wanted? Or will we declare and stand on our commitment to the healthy life style we deserve?

The good news is that each one of us is capable of making that choice; and once we are truly committed the how-to will not be a problem. Archimedes said: *give me a fulcrum and a sufficiently long lever and I will move the world*. When it comes to real and lasting change, the pain of the misery, and the vision of the life we were meant to have, act as the most effective levers. But daily, renewed commitment is the fulcrum without which no lever can be effective. Without it, we will be wasting our time (might as well stay miserable and like it). With it, we can move our world.

Sure, commitment can wane and fade away if we don't renew it daily. For this reason, we need *accountability* and *support*. Like their counterparts in the field of chemical dependency, groups such as *Overeaters Anonymous*, *Weight Watchers* and others in the recovery community (like Robert's circle of committed friends) understand the importance of this. They provide the needed support and encouragement; they remind us of our need for ongoing commitment; they give us the opportunity to learn and reap hope and courage from the lives of others; they hold us accountable to remain true to ourselves and transparent to one another; and they provide us with the necessary steps and tools to walk the path of victory and freedom from our addictions.

(Unfortunately, some of these accountability groups have no clear or workable understanding of the importance of the glycemic index, with the result of often endorsing diets that simply focus on calories. Counting calories can easily lead to the vicious cycle of dieting that often results in inadequate nutrition and inevitable rebound weight gain that is so prevalent in our weight and dieting conscious society. *Instead, the support and accountability these recovery groups provide must be aimed at promoting our commitment to a life-altering and sustainable style of healthy eating and proper exercise, as well as psychological and spiritual growth*.)

Now, let us look at the deeper problem that plagues the lives of those of us who are more like Kate or Mary. We know that the mental and emotional walls that keep us from changing, that keep us from personal freedom, are rooted deeply in a distorted self-image or self-concept. *It is not who we are, but who we believe we are that keeps us enslaved*. And, in these cases, it is the *internalized standard of the ideal body* that becomes our slave master and puppeteer.

As children we were all by nature vulnerable. When we were very young, we didn't have the capacity to accurately distinguish between fact and fallacy. Anything our caregivers (or any powerful significant other) told us about ourselves—through verbal and, especially, non-verbal language—was accepted without question.

These false reflections of ourselves, of how we saw ourselves through the eyes of those powerful others in our lives, were usually framed in terms of our bodies. Seemingly harmless appraisals that went deep and cut into our sense of self: *I see you haven't been working out. You're getting fat! Ah, you've finally lost weight! Wow, you're really ripped (or buff)! That looks terrible on you! You need to lose that double chin. Your thighs are too thick. Here, why don't you try this on your face to hide those wrinkles?*

Familiar?

Note that even though some messages may sound positive and affirming on the surface, the deeper message to the child may be that he or she is valued by a false standard: by how we look, rather than who we are. Better affirming statements would be: You are a kind, considerate person. *You are a good friend. You are trustworthy...loving...courageous...* Imagine a family, community, or society where one's external appearance is not the center of conversation, never an issue. Imagine what it would be like for people to see, appreciate and address one another in terms of the inner person. *Health would be a valid issue, not looks. The correction of bad habits or self-defeating patterns would be motivated by concern for the other person's health and well-being, and aimed at helping the person be free and fulfilled, rather than looking thinner, prettier, more buff, etc.* Utopian? Some may think so, but real and sustainable change comes from the inside out and is futile without a healthy self-identity.

Wanting to please others, to be accepted and admired by others, we have innocently allowed our bodies to become a central part of our self-image. This, of course, opened us up for all kinds of body image distortions. The essence of these distortions can be boiled down to a *my-body-is-not-acceptable* message, which translates into *I-am-not-good-enough.* Instead of a true image of ourselves—of who we truly are as individuals, of what truly gives us value as persons—we allowed a false, tyrannical standard to enter our minds and sit on the throne of self. And when we accepted this as children, we bit into the hook of this lie: *I have to fix myself, or be fixed, so that I can become worthy of love and acceptance.*

So, from early childhood, we embarked on this elusive quest after the mirage of an ideal body that would somehow bestow upon us the value and acceptance we have craved for most of our lives. And if you think we, as adults, have outgrown this, think again. The advertising industry is not so naïve; it knows our vulnerabilities and it constantly reminds us of this ideal, of how much we want it, and of how miserably we feel when we fail to attain it. All we have to do is to look and listen to the messages around us. Why do we spend so much time and energy buying and reading body beautiful self-help books, going to image remake seminars and workshops, buying the newest exercise gimmick?

As long as we believe this, and until we attain the ideal and are "fixed," we will continue to *feel* bad about ourselves. Defective. No one likes to feel this way. This is the reason we get caught up in the vicious cycle of doing anything and everything (compulsive dieting, severely restricting our food intake, purging, excessive exercising, and even chronic use of laxatives) to reshape our bodies to fit this *false ideal* of what it should be. This is pure tyranny.

There is no mistaking it; this ideal is an illusion and it is false because, even when some of us do attain it, it will never satisfy, it will never make us happy, it will never make us value or appreciate ourselves truly. We only have to look at the lives of the gorgeous, body-beautiful people who make up that exclusive club of movie idols so many in our society seem to revere. Honestly, how would we describe their lives as a whole if not shallow, unsatisfied, unhappy, unstable and just plain miserable?

Paradoxically, when we refuse to believe these negative and false appraisals of ourselves, and learn to value and love ourselves in our individual uniqueness, we will be motivated to care of and be good to ourselves. It is then that were are at the very best place for real and sustainable change that will keep us on the road to a healthy body, mind and spirit. (Personally, I base my self-worth and identity on my conviction that I am a child of a loving and merciful God, in whose image we were all created. No one can rob me of this, but we can certainly affirm each other in this. This realization fills and fulfills me, freeing me to love others who need my love, without having to play the I-will-love-you-if-you-love-me-and-accept-me game. Then the craving is to give and share, not to take and consume in order to fill the emptiness inside. On what or whom do you base your self-worth and identity?)

Let me try to make this as clear as I can to help dispel any lingering doubts and correct any residual misunderstandings. Accepting and loving the individual as a unique and worthy human being does not lead to the ignoring or condoning of self-defeating, harmful behavior, be it substance abuse, overeating, etc. On the contrary, it is because we value the individual that we are willing to go to the mat for him or her against that which is defeating and keeping that person enslaved.

Remember tough love? Unconditional love is central to this—anything else is a game we play with each other. Using a false ideal to motivate anyone to change comes straight out of the the-end-justifies-the-means school manual—and, believe me, the unfortunate students of that school fill the halls of the walking wounded.

In my practice, I have seen girls suffering from anorexia, looking like someone who came out of a concentration camp, emaciated, literally skin and bones. When asked what they see in the mirror, they invariable see themselves as being *fat*. These unfortunate girls are not seeing the true image of their bodies reflected in the mirror. They are seeing an internalized and incredibly distorted image of their body, an image that will forever fall short of the false ideal they are committed to attain, regardless of the cost, even to their deaths (like Alice).

Death by self-imposed starvation...Sounds extreme? But isn't this what we do to ourselves when we get caught up in the vicious cycle of compulsive dieting? Through the repeated insults of the self-imposed starvation common to most diet fads, our bodies become the victims to cumulative damage that hastens our death. We cannot afford to underestimate the tremendous emotional power of this *false ideal*.

Let me tell you an important secret: *we cannot change our feelings or emotions directly*. The illusion of the emotional fix is the illusion behind all forms of addiction (and the major reason why most of us relapse). The fact is that the more we try to fix, numb, or ignore our painful emotions, the more powerful these emotions become. And if we wait for our feelings to change before we commit ourselves and take the necessary steps to freedom, how long will we have to wait?

But here is another piece of good news: we can change the way we think and what we *do*—and, more importantly, *we can choose to believe or not to believe*. When we do change the things we can change, rather than controlling our lives, our emotions will eventually get in line and *follow our chosen path in life*. Don't let anyone tell you that you can't do it.

You can refuse to run for comfort to anything that ultimately harms you, but you have to be willing to *feel bad* for a while. (There is a price for freedom, but it is a price that is well worth it in the end.) Yes, all of us can *refuse* to believe in and follow that tyrannical *false ideal* (which we have allowed to rule our lives and emotions); we can *refuse* to fit the mold and instead give ourselves the opportunity to discover and appreciate who we are. It is a *process*—a road we walk—*not a leap*. It isn't about thinking fat or thinking thin; it's about thinking healthy and committing ourselves to do only that which is good for us, because we are learning to appreciate and love ourselves. If we want lasting victory, we have to be committed to the right cause.

It has been clearly demonstrated that the children with the healthiest self-concepts and, therefore, healthiest life styles by far are those who are raised in families that do not obsess or harp on food, eating, exercise and—especially—the way one looks. These are families with parents that teach by *example*, taking care of themselves at every level of our human existence (physical, mental-emotional, relational, spiritual...) *because* they value and love themselves in a healthy way. These children have parents whose life styles consistently reflect this attitude, parents who love and value each child in his or her individual, unique humanity (no comparing, no blueprints, no conditions to acceptance).

Unfortunately, no child can choose his or her parents or what family to be born into. *But each of us can learn to parent ourselves*. And we can learn to allow those who present us with a true reflection of our selves, who appreciate and value us (as they do themselves), who are serious about living a healthy life to the fullest, to become our surrogate family and our recovery community.

The tools for change are out there, just a phone call, a drive, or a click away. But *lasting change* is about thinking truly about ourselves; it's about looking beyond the body and discovering who we truly are; it's about appreciating and loving ourselves and taking good care of ourselves; and it is about having the hope and the courage to do so.

The Patino Diet

Introduction

You've probably tried a number of different diets before coming to us, but we all want to KNOW something works before we invest our time and energy into it. The PATINO DIET was developed by Dr. Patino for his own dietary needs, and unlike most of our competitors, Dr. Patino practices what he preaches... and has the body to show for it! At almost 60 years of age, Dr.Patino still has a healthy, trim body, with enough energy to spend on his private practice, business, hobbies, and growing family.

Dr. Patino built the PATINO DIET around four core concepts.

1. EASY TO FOLLOW AND UNDERSTAND
2. TASTY AND ENJOYABLE
3. SUSTAINABLE, PERMANENT WEIGHT LOSS
4. ADAPTABLE TO ANY DIETARY RESTRICTIONS

Dr. Patino has developed a breakthrough system based on the science of the Glycemic Index, enabling you to lose weight and develop a healthy lifestyle... permanently! In fact, the PATINO DIET isn't really a diet at all, but a lifestyle change that enables you to choose WHAT you want to eat, WHEN you want to eat. If you love food, hate being told what to eat and when, then you have come to the right place.

The PATINO DIET is divided into two simple stages.

STAGE 1 *Lifestyle* CHANGE

In Stage 1, we introduce you to the PATINO DIET and the healthy, delicious foods that will become the core of your new dietary lifestyle. "The Age of Globesity: Entering the Perfect Storm" includes a meal plan for your first month, as well as dozens of recipes to spice up your dinner table. The goal is to teach you what you can and can not eat, as well as guiding you into a healthy and maintenance free life style that sheds weight automatically! For most people, you will lose 10 to 15 pd. in the first few weeks!

You'll stay in Stage 1 for about a month, and then move to Stage 2.

STAGE 2 *Lifestyle* MAINTENANCE

By now, you should have an understanding of the PATINO DIET and a low Glycemic Index dietary plan, so the training wheels come off. You are free to create your own dietary plan incorporating our teachings, and are given the room for "cheat days" where you can eat whatever you want! This program is NOT built for a quick fix, but to create a daily lifestyle that burns fat and keeps you at your ideal weight forever!

That's it. No complicated meal plans, no crazy carb counting. The PATINO DIET educates you to make the RIGHT decisions for a healthy, balanced lifestyle, and leaves the decisions up to you on how you construct your culinary schedule.

Stage One

So you've decided to take the first steps toward a healthier you? Congratulations! We have included a meal plan regiment with a month of tasty and nutritious selections, but the primary goal is for you to educate yourself. You need to learn what foods are good for you, and what foods to avoid.

Let's list off a few items from the good and bad lists, so you can see an idea of what is required.

GOOD FOR YOU (low GI)	BAD FOR YOU (high GI)
• Most Meats (lean cuts)	• Potatoes & Starches
• Most Fruit	• Most Rice
• Most Vegetables	• Most Bread
• Most Beans	• Most Pasta
• Most Nuts	• Sugar
	• Most Processed Foods

Of course, this is a highly simplified list, but you can always look up the individual GI and GL values for any particular food in the index at the back of the book.

During stage 1, we take all the guess work out of your diet, providing you with full meal plans and recipes to get you started. By the end of your meal plans, you should have a healthy understanding of what you can and can not eat. It is this education that will provide you with your most potent weapon in fighting fat, for you will be able to make educated decisions on what you can and can not allow into your dietary regiment.

Most people stay in Stage 1 for about a month, and then move on to Stage 2, but you can alter this if you have not quite reached your goals.

30 Day Meal Plan

And now we get to the good part. The FOOD! The sad truth is that most dieters have been misled into believing that a healthy diet is a bland diet. As you will see as you read through Stage One's meal plans, that is far from the case for the PATINO DIET!

We believe that it is imperative that a diet be worth eating on the food's own merit and tastiness, not just for how healthy it might be. But don't take our word for it, take look for yourself. We guarantee your mouth will be watering too!

If you find that a particular day's menu doesn't appeal to you, just replace it with an item you found scrumptious. We don't require that you follow the plans to the letter, just that you only eat from the approved recipes listed in the following sections.

Many of our delicious recipes were donated by local restaurants in the Greater Detroit area, so if you happen to live nearby, feel free to stop by and check out their cuisine in person. We have included more information on those restaurants in the Contributor section, so make sure to check it out!

Day 1

Breakfast
- ❖ **Smoothie** (your choice, from page 225)
- ❖ **Fruit** (your choice, be wary of tropical varieties)

Morning Snack
- ❖ Choose a snack from the Snack section on page 241.

Lunch
- ❖ **BLT Lettuce Wrap**
- ❖ **Coleslaw** (unsweetened, no sugar added)

Afternoon Snack
- ❖ Choose a snack from the Snack section on page 241.

Dinner
- ❖ **Flank Steak**
- ❖ **Peanut Kale Salad**
- ❖ **Vegetable** (steamed or grilled, preferably green)

Dessert
- ❖ Choose a dessert from the Dessert section on page 244.

Day 2

Breakfast
- ❖ **Spinach and Cheese Omelet**
- ❖ **Yogurt** (with or without fruit, unsweetened)

Morning Snack
- ❖ Choose a snack from the Snack section on page 241.

Lunch
- ❖ **Gruyere Cheese Caesar Salad**
- ❖ **Applesauce** (unsweetened)

Afternoon Snack
- ❖ Choose a snack from the Snack section on page 241.

Dinner
- ❖ **Halibut in Herbs and Oil**
- ❖ **Crab and Avocado with Tomato**
- ❖ **Vegetable** (steamed or grilled, preferably green)

Dessert
- ❖ Choose a dessert from the Dessert section on page 244.

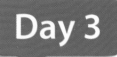

Day 3

Breakfast
❖ **Baked Eggs and Bacon**
❖ **Low GI Bread** (sourdough, rye, pumpernickel, etc.)

Morning Snack
❖ Choose a snack from the Snack section on page 241.

Lunch
❖ **Garden Salad with Grilled Chicken**
❖ **Vegetables** (raw, with or without dipping sauce)

Afternoon Snack
❖ Choose a snack from the Snack section on page 241.

Dinner
❖ **Rack of Lamb**
❖ **Farro Salad with Whipped Goa Cheese**
❖ **Vegetable** (steamed or grilled, preferably green)

Dessert
❖ Choose a dessert from the Dessert section on page 244.

Day 4

Breakfast
- ❖ **Smoothie** (your choice, from page 225)
- ❖ **Fruit** (your choice, be wary of tropical varieties)

Morning Snack
- ❖ Choose a snack from the Snack section on page 241.

Lunch
- ❖ **Lettuce Roll Up** (your choice of meat)
- ❖ **Fruit** (your choice, be wary of tropical varieties)

Afternoon Snack
- ❖ Choose a snack from the Snack section on page 241.

Dinner
- ❖ **Spicy Sausage and Ground Beef Meatballs**
- ❖ **Celery, Walnut and Lemon Thyme Salad**
- ❖ **Vegetable** (steamed or grilled, preferably green)

Dessert
- ❖ Choose a dessert from the Dessert section on page 244.

Day 5

Breakfast
- ❖ **Steel Cut Oatmeal with Sliced Apples and Cinnamon**
- ❖ **Yogurt** (with or without fruit, unsweetened)

Morning Snack
- ❖ Choose a snack from the Snack section on page 241.

Lunch
- ❖ **Mild Lamb Stew**
- ❖ **Hummus with Low GI Pita Crisps**

Afternoon Snack
- ❖ Choose a snack from the Snack section on page 241.

Dinner
- ❖ **Moroccan Roasted Chicken**
- ❖ **Cheddar Soup**
- ❖ **Vegetable** (steamed or grilled, preferably green)

Dessert
- ❖ Choose a dessert from the Dessert section on page 244.

Day 6

Breakfast
- ❖ **Breakfast Burrito**
- ❖ **Veggie Hash**

Morning Snack
- ❖ Choose a snack from the Snack section on page 241.

Lunch
- ❖ **Burger** (wrapped in lettuce, with or without cheese)
- ❖ **Fruit** (your choice, be wary of tropical varieties)

Afternoon Snack
- ❖ Choose a snack from the Snack section on page 241.

Dinner
- ❖ **Grilled Salmon with Cucumber Basil**
- ❖ **Cucumber Salad**
- ❖ **Vegetable** (steamed or grilled, preferably green)

Dessert
- ❖ Choose a dessert from the Dessert section on page 244.

Day 7

Breakfast

- ❖ **Faux French Toast**
- ❖ **Fruit** (your choice, be wary of tropical varieties)

Morning Snack

- ❖ Choose a snack from the Snack section on page 241.

Lunch

- ❖ **Tuna and Avocado Salad**
- ❖ **Fruit** (your choice, be wary of tropical varieties)

Afternoon Snack

- ❖ Choose a snack from the Snack section on page 241.

Dinner

- ❖ **Seared Tuna Sashimi**
- ❖ **Spinach Salad**
- ❖ **Vegetable** (steamed or grilled, preferably green)

Dessert

- ❖ Choose a dessert from the Dessert section on page 244.

Day 8

Breakfast
* **Smoothie** (your choice, from page 225)
* **Fruit** (your choice, be wary of tropical varieties)

Morning Snack
* Choose a snack from the Snack section on page 241.

Lunch
* **Spicy Chicken with Boiled Eggs**
* **Coleslaw** (unsweetened, no sugar added)

Afternoon Snack
* Choose a snack from the Snack section on page 241.

Dinner
* **Tuscan Steak with Sauce Ammoglio**
* **Marinated Kale Salad**
* **Vegetable** (steamed or grilled, preferably green)

Dessert
* Choose a dessert from the Dessert section on page 244.

Day 9

Breakfast
- ❖ **Scrambled Eggs with Gruyere and Salmon**
- ❖ **Low GI Bread** (sourdough, rye, pumpernickel, etc.)

Morning Snack
- ❖ Choose a snack from the Snack section on page 241.

Lunch
- ❖ **Peanut Kale Salad** (with grilled chicken)
- ❖ **Snackin' Fries**

Afternoon Snack
- ❖ Choose a snack from the Snack section on page 241.

Dinner
- ❖ **Chicken with Rosemary and Garlic**
- ❖ **Duck Salad**
- ❖ **Vegetable** (steamed or grilled, preferably green)

Dessert
- ❖ Choose a dessert from the Dessert section on page 244.

Day 10

Breakfast
❖ **Strawberry Crepes**
❖ **Yogurt** (with or without fruit, unsweetened)

Morning Snack
❖ Choose a snack from the Snack section on page 241.

Lunch
❖ **Garden Salad with Grilled Chicken**
❖ **Vegetables** (raw, with or without dipping sauce)

Afternoon Snack
❖ Choose a snack from the Snack section on page 241.

Dinner
❖ **Tuscan Veal with Lemon and Mushrooms**
❖ **Spinach Salad**
❖ **Vegetable** (steamed or grilled, preferably green)

Dessert
❖ Choose a dessert from the Dessert section on page 244.

Day 11

Breakfast
- ❖ **Smoothie** (your choice, from page 225)
- ❖ **Fruit** (your choice, be wary of tropical varieties)

Morning Snack
- ❖ Choose a snack from the Snack section on page 241.

Lunch
- ❖ **Reuben Sandwich** (on rye bread)
- ❖ **Coleslaw** (unsweetened, no sugar added)

Afternoon Snack
- ❖ Choose a snack from the Snack section on page 241.

Dinner
- ❖ **Mojo Pork Roast**
- ❖ **Crab and Avocado with Tomato**
- ❖ **Vegetable** (steamed or grilled, preferably green)

Dessert
- ❖ Choose a dessert from the Dessert section on page 244.

Day 12

Breakfast
❖ **Ham and Cheese Omelet**
❖ **Fruit** (your choice, be wary of tropical varieties)

Morning Snack
❖ Choose a snack from the Snack section on page 241.

Lunch
❖ **Steak Bites**
❖ **Coleslaw** (unsweetened, no sugar added)

Afternoon Snack
❖ Choose a snack from the Snack section on page 241.

Dinner
❖ **Filet Mignon with Portobello Sauce**
❖ **White Truffle Butternut Squash Soup**
❖ **Vegetable** (steamed or grilled, preferably green)

Dessert
❖ Choose a dessert from the Dessert section on page 244.

Day 13

Breakfast
- ❖ **Breakfast Burrito**
- ❖ **Yogurt** (with or without fruit, unsweetened)

Morning Snack
- ❖ Choose a snack from the Snack section on page 241.

Lunch
- ❖ **Lettuce Roll Up** (your choice of meat)
- ❖ **Fruit** (your choice, be wary of tropical varieties)

Afternoon Snack
- ❖ Choose a snack from the Snack section on page 241.

Dinner
- ❖ **Shrimp with Rosemary and Arugula**
- ❖ **Ethiopian Salad**
- ❖ **Vegetable** (steamed or grilled, preferably green)

Dessert
- ❖ Choose a dessert from the Dessert section on page 244.

Day 14

Breakfast
❖ **Bacon and Eggs**
❖ **Low GI Bread** (sourdough, rye, pumpernickel, etc.)

Morning Snack
❖ Choose a snack from the Snack section on page 241.

Lunch
❖ **BLT Lettuce Wrap**
❖ **Fruit** (your choice, be wary of tropical varieties)

Afternoon Snack
❖ Choose a snack from the Snack section on page 241.

Dinner
❖ **Spicy Beef**
❖ **Yellow Split Peas**
❖ **Vegetable** (steamed or grilled, preferably green)

Dessert
❖ Choose a dessert from the Dessert section on page 244.

Day 15

Breakfast
- ❖ **Smoothie** (your choice, from page 225)
- ❖ **Fruit** (your choice, be wary of tropical varieties)

Morning Snack
- ❖ Choose a snack from the Snack section on page 241.

Lunch
- ❖ **Caesar Salad with Grilled Chicken** (no croutons)
- ❖ **Coleslaw** (unsweetened, no sugar added)

Afternoon Snack
- ❖ Choose a snack from the Snack section on page 241.

Dinner
- ❖ **Swordfish 'Tireno'**
- ❖ **Celery, Walnut and Lemon Thyme Salad**
- ❖ **Vegetable** (steamed or grilled, preferably green)

Dessert
- ❖ Choose a dessert from the Dessert section on page 244.

Day 16

Breakfast
- ❖ **Breakfast Burrito**
- ❖ **Veggie Hash**

Morning Snack
- ❖ Choose a snack from the Snack section on page 241.

Lunch
- ❖ **Cocoa/Cinnamon/Chili Beef Carpaccio**
- ❖ **Fruit** (your choice, be wary of tropical varieties)

Afternoon Snack
- ❖ Choose a snack from the Snack section on page 241.

Dinner
- ❖ **Seared Scallops with Oxtail Ragu**
- ❖ **Tofu and Avocado Timbale**
- ❖ **Vegetable** (steamed or grilled, preferably green)

Dessert
- ❖ Choose a dessert from the Dessert section on page 244.

Day 17

Breakfast
- ❖ **Steel Cut Oatmeal Pancakes with Yogurt and Fruit**
- ❖ **Fruit** (your choice, be wary of tropical varieties)

Morning Snack
- ❖ Choose a snack from the Snack section on page 241.

Lunch
- ❖ **Ham Rolls with Cream Cheese and Chives**
- ❖ **Watermelon Gazpacho**

Afternoon Snack
- ❖ Choose a snack from the Snack section on page 241.

Dinner
- ❖ **Braised Lamb Shanks**
- ❖ **Zucchini Carpaccio**
- ❖ **Vegetable** (steamed or grilled, preferably green)

Dessert
- ❖ Choose a dessert from the Dessert section on page 244.

Day 18

Breakfast
- ❖ **Strawberry Crepes**
- ❖ **Low GI Bread** (sourdough, rye, pumpernickel, etc.)

Morning Snack
- ❖ Choose a snack from the Snack section on page 241.

Lunch
- ❖ **Seared Tuna Sashimi**
- ❖ **Fruit** (your choice, be wary of tropical varieties)

Afternoon Snack
- ❖ Choose a snack from the Snack section on page 241.

Dinner
- ❖ **Sea Scallops in a Sherry Sauce**
- ❖ **Ethiopian Salad**
- ❖ **Vegetable** (steamed or grilled, preferably green)

Dessert
- ❖ Choose a dessert from the Dessert section on page 244.

Day 19

Breakfast
- ❖ **Smoothie** (your choice, from page 225)
- ❖ **Fruit** (your choice, be wary of tropical varieties)

Morning Snack
- ❖ Choose a snack from the Snack section on page 241.

Lunch
- ❖ **Chicken with Rosemary and Garlic**
- ❖ **Coleslaw** (unsweetened, no sugar added)

Afternoon Snack
- ❖ Choose a snack from the Snack section on page 241.

Dinner
- ❖ **Mediterranean Grouper**
- ❖ **White Truffle Butternut Squash Soup**
- ❖ **Vegetable** (steamed or grilled, preferably green)

Dessert
- ❖ Choose a dessert from the Dessert section on page 244.

Day 20

Breakfast
❖ **Faux French Toast**
❖ **Fruit** (your choice, be wary of tropical varieties)

Morning Snack
❖ Choose a snack from the Snack section on page 241.

Lunch
❖ **Garden Salad with Grilled Steak**
❖ **Fruit** (your choice, be wary of tropical varieties)

Afternoon Snack
❖ Choose a snack from the Snack section on page 241.

Dinner
❖ **Meatloaf**
❖ **Cucumber Salad**
❖ **Vegetable** (steamed or grilled, preferably green)

Dessert
❖ Choose a dessert from the Dessert section on page 244.

Day 21

Breakfast

- ❖ **Spinach and Cheese Omelet**
- ❖ **Yogurt** (with or without fruit, unsweetened)

Morning Snack

- ❖ Choose a snack from the Snack section on page 241.

Lunch

- ❖ **Garden Salad with Grilled Chicken**
- ❖ **Snackin' Fries**

Afternoon Snack

- ❖ Choose a snack from the Snack section on page 241.

Dinner

- ❖ **Chicken and Artichokes**
- ❖ **Marinated Kale Salad**
- ❖ **Vegetable** (steamed or grilled, preferably green)

Dessert

- ❖ Choose a dessert from the Dessert section on page 244.

Day 22

Breakfast
- ❖ **Garden Omelet**
- ❖ **Veggie Hash**

Morning Snack
- ❖ Choose a snack from the Snack section on page 241.

Lunch
- ❖ **Bleu Cheese Steak Salad**
- ❖ **Fruit** (your choice, be wary of tropical varieties)

Afternoon Snack
- ❖ Choose a snack from the Snack section on page 241.

Dinner
- ❖ **Mojo Pork Roast**
- ❖ **Marinara Primavera**
- ❖ **Vegetable** (steamed or grilled, preferably green)

Dessert
- ❖ Choose a dessert from the Dessert section on page 244.

Day 23

Breakfast
❖ **Smoothie** (your choice, from page 225)
❖ **Fruit** (your choice, be wary of tropical varieties)

Morning Snack
❖ Choose a snack from the Snack section on page 241.

Lunch
❖ **Lettuce Roll Up** (your choice of meat)
❖ **Fruit** (your choice, be wary of tropical varieties)

Afternoon Snack
❖ Choose a snack from the Snack section on page 241.

Dinner
❖ **Rack of Lamb**
❖ **White Truffle Butternut Squash Soup**
❖ **Vegetable** (steamed or grilled, preferably green)

Dessert
❖ Choose a dessert from the Dessert section on page 244.

Day 24

Breakfast
- ❖ **Steel Cut Oatmeal Pancakes with Yogurt and Fruit**
- ❖ **Low GI Bread** (sourdough, rye, pumpernickel, etc.)

Morning Snack
- ❖ Choose a snack from the Snack section on page 241.

Lunch
- ❖ **Meatloaf**
- ❖ **Coleslaw** (unsweetened, no sugar added)

Afternoon Snack
- ❖ Choose a snack from the Snack section on page 241.

Dinner
- ❖ **Island BBQ Ribs**
- ❖ **Celery, Walnut and Lemon Thyme Salad**
- ❖ **Vegetable** (steamed or grilled, preferably green)

Dessert
- ❖ Choose a dessert from the Dessert section on page 244.

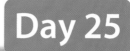

Day 25

Breakfast
- ❖ **Baked Eggs and Bacon**
- ❖ **Fruit** (your choice, be wary of tropical varieties)

Morning Snack
- ❖ Choose a snack from the Snack section on page 241.

Lunch
- ❖ **Greek Salad with Chicken**
- ❖ **Fruit** (your choice, be wary of tropical varieties)

Afternoon Snack
- ❖ Choose a snack from the Snack section on page 241.

Dinner
- ❖ **Flank Steak**
- ❖ **Broccoli and Cheese Soup**
- ❖ **Vegetable** (steamed or grilled, preferably green)

Dessert
- ❖ Choose a dessert from the Dessert section on page 244.

Day 26

Breakfast
❖ **Smoothie** (your choice, from page 225)
❖ **Fruit** (your choice, be wary of tropical varieties)

Morning Snack
❖ Choose a snack from the Snack section on page 241.

Lunch
❖ **Spicy Beef**
❖ **Fruit** (your choice, be wary of tropical varieties)

Afternoon Snack
❖ Choose a snack from the Snack section on page 241.

Dinner
❖ **Mediterranean Grouper**
❖ **Cucumber Salad**
❖ **Vegetable** (steamed or grilled, preferably green)

Dessert
❖ Choose a dessert from the Dessert section on page 244.

Day 27

Breakfast
- ❖ **Breakfast Burrito**
- ❖ **Yogurt** (with or without fruit, unsweetened)

Morning Snack
- ❖ Choose a snack from the Snack section on page 241.

Lunch
- ❖ **Spinach and Strawberry Salad**
- ❖ **Fruit** (your choice, be wary of tropical varieties)

Afternoon Snack
- ❖ Choose a snack from the Snack section on page 241.

Dinner
- ❖ **Filet Mignon with Portobello Sauce**
- ❖ **Ethiopian Salad**
- ❖ **Vegetable** (steamed or grilled, preferably green)

Dessert
- ❖ Choose a dessert from the Dessert section on page 244.

Day 28

Breakfast
- ❖ **Scrambled Eggs with Gruyere and Salmon**
- ❖ **Low GI Bread** (sourdough, rye, pumpernickel, etc.)

Morning Snack
- ❖ Choose a snack from the Snack section on page 241.

Lunch
- ❖ **Tandoori Chicken Wings**
- ❖ **Fruit** (your choice, be wary of tropical varieties)

Afternoon Snack
- ❖ Choose a snack from the Snack section on page 241.

Dinner
- ❖ **Mojo Pork Roast**
- ❖ **Ethiopian Salad**
- ❖ **Vegetable** (steamed or grilled, preferably green)

Dessert
- ❖ Choose a dessert from the Dessert section on page 244.

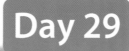

Day 29

Breakfast
- ❖ **Strawberry Crepes**
- ❖ **Fruit** (your choice, be wary of tropical varieties)

Morning Snack
- ❖ Choose a snack from the Snack section on page 241.

Lunch
- ❖ **Lettuce Wraps** (meat of choice)
- ❖ **Coleslaw** (unsweetened, no sugar added)

Afternoon Snack
- ❖ Choose a snack from the Snack section on page 241.

Dinner
- ❖ **Mediterranean Sea Bass**
- ❖ **Crab and Avocado with Tomato**
- ❖ **Vegetable** (steamed or grilled, preferably green)

Dessert
- ❖ Choose a dessert from the Dessert section on page 244.

Day 30

Breakfast
- ❖ **Smoothie** (your choice, from page 225)
- ❖ **Fruit** (your choice, be wary of tropical varieties)

Morning Snack
- ❖ Choose a snack from the Snack section on page 241.

Lunch
- ❖ **Ham Rolls with Cream Cheese and Chives**
- ❖ **Fruit** (your choice, be wary of tropical varieties)

Afternoon Snack
- ❖ Choose a snack from the Snack section on page 241.

Dinner
- ❖ **Grilled Salmon 'Tireno'**
- ❖ **Spinach Salad**
- ❖ **Vegetable** (steamed or grilled, preferably green)

Dessert
- ❖ Choose a dessert from the Dessert section on page 244.

Stage Two

So you've reached your target weight, and things are looking up. With most diets, people simply go back to the way they used to eat, and eventually put those pounds right back on. This is not like those diets, and it is the primary reason we call the PATINO DIET a lifestyle change. We are not just teaching you how to lose a few pounds, we are showing how to KEEP that weight off... forever!

By now, you should have a firm understanding of how the Glycemic Index impacts your body. You should know what foods you can, and even more importantly, can **not** eat. You should have already overcome the bulk of your cravings for sugar and processed food, and be comfortable with your dieting regiment. In short, you have all the ingredients to keep yourself lean, thin, and healthy... you just have to stick with it!

You have, however, earned yourself a little wiggle room. You can and probably should have a cheat day every week or two, where you indulge in some of the high GI items you miss in your daily diet. As long as you keep those indulgences moderate and spread out over your cheat day, they should have no effect on your overall health. But please exercise caution, as some people find the ability to cheat in their regiment a slippery slope.

The key to success in the last stage of the PATINO DIET is consistency. You have the knowledge and the tools to make the right decisions, so do it!

Eating Out

Dining out scares many dieters, but if you have followed the precepts taught to you throughout this book, you should be prepared to order with confidence. Almost every restaurant has options that are friendly to a conscientious eater, but make certain to stay disciplined when ordering. You should know what to eat; do not break your regiment for an indulgence that will set you back!

To simplify the process, we have prepared a simple set of guidelines to keep in mind while dining out. They will assist you in making the right decisions, and help keep you on track for your dietary and health goals.

1. **Skip the bread basket** (unless your fellow diners require it).

Many times, that initial temptation is the one that pushes us into breaking our regiment. Avoid it entirely by removing it from the equation, when possible.

2. **Order a healthy soup or salad to start.**

Here in the US, portion sizes have been bloated out of control. Unfortunately, it takes 20 to 30 minutes for our stomachs to even recognize that they are full, which creates a scenario where American eaters have a tendency to overeat before they even have a chance to recognize how full they really are! You can avoid this by starting your meal with a healthy soup or salad, and thus shortening the time it takes for your brain to recognize how full you really are when the main entrée arrives.

3. Make protein the star of your meal.

Almost every restaurant in the US has several option for a protein rich diet, whether your tastes are for meat, pork, chicken, or seafood. Let the bulk of your appetite be satiated here, and avoid any carb heavy selections.

As a side note to a protein heavy entrée, please refrain from any fried foods. While Olive Oil can be a healthy addition of fat to your regiment, restaurants rarely fry their food in it. Grilled, seared, roasted, broiled, steamed, baked, even sautéed can be fine, but you should do your best to avoid the heavy saturated fats that most fried foods are cooked in.

4. Try asking for a lettuce wrap instead of bread.

Many restaurants will wrap a sandwich in lettuce instead of bread, if it is requested. This creates a healthy alternative to loading up on a high GI carbs in a sandwich or sub. A few chains have even established this as a healthy alternative on their menus, like Jimmy John's "Unwich".

5. No potatoes, rice, or pasta!

You should already be quite familiar with the dangers of these particular food groups at this stage, but it bears reminding. There are healthy alternatives for rice and pasta that have decent GI/GL responses, but you will almost never find them in a restaurant. As such, it is better to completely avoid the temptation. Ask for a double order of veggies or a salad instead!

6. Beware the sauces!

It is difficult, if not impossible, to know the sugar and health content of any particular sauce or dressing. As such, order it on the side and make the decision on how much (if any) that you will use in your meal. When possible, skip the sauce if you can.

In regards to salad dressings, if they do not offer a sugar free option just ask for olive oil, vinegar, or lemon wedges. They can spice up a salad quite nicely with little to no effect on your GI.

7. Say NO to desert.

There are plenty of healthy deserts from you to choose from, but you will find very few of them out at a restaurant. Treat yourself to something when you get home, or save it for your cheat day.

8. Do not be afraid to grab a doggy bag!

Portion control is out of control, especially here in the US. If you find yourself satisfied before finishing your meal, take it home and enjoy it later. The outdated and unhealthy mentality that you must "finish everything on your plate" only works to encourage over-eating and indulgence.

With these simple tips, you should be well on your way to ordering a healthy meal at just about any establishment. Enjoy!

RECIPES

Entrees

- ❖ Braised Lamb Shanks
- ❖ Chicken and Artichokes
- ❖ Filet Mignon with Portobello Sauce
- ❖ Flank Steak
- ❖ Grilled Salmon with Cucumber Basil
- ❖ Grilled Salmon 'Tireno'
- ❖ Halibut in Herbs & Oil
- ❖ Island BBQ Ribs
- ❖ Mediterranean Grouper
- ❖ Mediterranean Sea Bass
- ❖ Mojo Pork Roast
- ❖ Moroccan Roasted Chicken
- ❖ Rack of Lamb
- ❖ Sea Scallops in a Sherry Sauce
- ❖ Seared Scallops with Oxtail Ragu
- ❖ Shrimp with Rosemary & Arugula
- ❖ Spicy Sausage & Ground Beef Meatballs
- ❖ Spicy Yellow Split Peas
- ❖ Swordfish 'Tireno'
- ❖ Tuscan Steak with Sauce Ammoglio
- ❖ Tuscan Veal with Lemon & Mushrooms

Braised Lamb Shanks

Ingredients:

- 4 lamb shanks, ~ 1 pd. each (rinsed and patted dry)
- ½ cup of low carb flour
- 2 tbsp. of butter or olive oil
- sea salt and fresh ground pepper (to taste)
- 1 onion (peeled and chopped)
- 1 large carrot (chopped)
- 2 celery stalks (chopped)
- 1 small (about ½ cup) fennel pod (cored and chopped)
- ½ tsp. *srircha* (hotsauce)
- 1 28 oz. can of tomatoes (diced with juice)
- 1 cup of red wine
- 4 large garlic cloves (peeled and roughly chopped)
- 2 tbsp. fresh rosemary (roughly chopped)
- 1 lemon (zest and juice)
- 2 tsp. of cardamom
- 1 tsp. of thyme (minced)

Preparation:

1. Dredge the shanks in the flour 2 at a time, shaking off any excess.
2. Add salt and pepper.
3. Melt 1 tbsp. of butter or oil in a cast-iron or sauté pan large enough to accommodate 2 shanks at a time.
4. Over medium-high to high heat, brown 2 shanks at a time, about 2 minutes a side or a total of 8 minutes.
5. Transfer to an oven proof container large enough to accommodate all of the shanks.
6. Repeat steps 3 – 5 with the remaining 2 shanks.
7. Add the chopped onion, carrot, celery, fennel and garlic to the same pan, using an additional tbsp. of fat if necessary.
8. Season with salt and pepper.
9. Sauté the vegetables for about 5 minutes, just until they soften and wilt, being careful not to brown.
10. Remove the pan from the heat and add the remaining ingredients, stirring to incorporate into the vegetables.
11. Transfer the vegetables to the baking dish
12. Cook at 350 degrees for about 1 ½ hours, until just tender.
    Note: shanks are best made a day ahead and reheated in the oven

Recipe donated by **Café Muse** of Royal Oak, MI

Chicken and Artichokes

Ingredients:

- 1 pd. of skinless chicken breast
- 6 oz. of marinated artichoke hearts
- 1 tbsp. of parmesan cheese
- black pepper

Preparation:

1. Coat a nonstick pan or skillet with non-stick cooking spray.
2. Sauté the chicken breast.
3. Drain artichoke hearts and add to pan with chicken.
4. Remove from pan and place on plate.
5. Sprinkle parmesan cheese on top.
6. Add black pepper (to taste).

Filet Mignon with Portobello Sauce

Ingredients:

- 4 filet mignon steaks
- 2 large portobello mushrooms (halved and sliced)
- 8 green onions cut into 1 inch pieces
- ⅓ cup of reduced sodium beef broth
- 2 tbsp. of red wine
- 1 tbsp. of butter
- 1 tsp. of olive oil
- ¼ tsp. of black pepper

Preparation:

1. Mix olive oil and pepper, then baste both sides of the steaks.
2. Heat a pan to medium heat and add butter, sauté mushrooms and onions until tender.
3. Add beef broth and red wine to pan, than bring to a boil.
4. Remove sauce from heat and set aside.
5. Grill steaks over medium heat until desired doneness, turning once halfway through grilling.
6. When done, slice steak thin and smother with the sauté sauce.

Flank Steak

Ingredients:

- 1 pd. of flank steak
- Italian salad dressing
- 2 tbsp. of olive oil
- 1 tbsp. of lemon juice

Preparation:

1. Spread Italian dressing mix over one side of the steak.
2. Roll up the steak like a crescent roll, with the seasoned side facing inward. Tie the steak together with a string and place in a baking pan.
3. Spread the remaining mix across the exterior of the rolled steak.
4. Cover the steak with cellophane wrap and refrigerate overnight.
5. Grill until desired doneness, turning frequently.
6. Remove string and lay steak flat on the grill, searing steak on both sides.

Italian Dressing

Ingredients:

- 2 cups of olive oil
- ¼ cup of lemon juice
- ¼ cup of balsamic vinegar
- 1 tsp. of salt
- 1 tsp. of sugar substitute
- 1.2 tsp. of oregano, dried
- ½ tsp. of thyme, ground
- ½ tsp. of onion powder
- 2 garlic cloves, crushed

Preparation:

1. Vigorously mix all ingredients in covered container.
2. Refrigerate overnight and after use.

Grilled Salmon with Cucumber Basil

Ingredients:

- 2 pd. of fresh wild caught salmon (cut into four servings)
- 2 English cucumbers
- 1 large daikon radish
- fresh basil
- 4 tbsp. of lime juice
- 1 tbsp. of agave nectar
- 6 tbsp. of grape seed oil
- 4-8 rice paper wrappers
- salt and pepper (to taste)

Preparation:

1. Start by heating the grill to medium high heat.
2. Brush the salmon with oil, season with salt and pepper.
3. Using a mandolin slicer, cut 1 cucumber into match stick shaped pieces. *Note: Only use the outside of the cucumber, reserve the inside of the cucumber for the broth.*
4. Use the same technique with the entire daikon radish.
5. In a separate bowl combine the lime juice, agave nectar, and oil. Whisk together and season with salt and pepper.
6. Toss in the matchstick cut veggies.
7. Using cold water, submerge the rice paper for approximately 30 seconds. Lay out on flat service. Add some of the vegetable mix to the center of each rice paper, then fold corners over the vegetables.
8. Roll the rice paper around the vegetable mix.
9. Repeat process for the remaining rice papers.
10. In a blender or juicer, puree the remaining cucumber till smooth and liquefied. Add 6 basil leaves and a pinch of salt.
11. Continue to mix till smooth.
12. Grill salmon till desired doneness (we recommend medium).

Presentation:

1. Place grilled salmon on plate side by side with one fresh roll.
2. Spoon the cucumber broth liberally over each salmon and fresh roll.

Recipe Donated by **Cliff Bells** of Detroit, MI

Grilled Salmon 'Tireno'

Salmone 'Tireno' Alle Griglia

Ingredients:

- 2 cups of pesto oil (for marinating)
- ⅔ cup of extra virgin olive oil
- 2 tsp. of garlic, minced
- 3 cups of roma tomatoes, coarsely chopped
- 1 tsp. of salt
- 1 cup of dry white wine
- ½ cup of basil, finely chopped

- 2 basil sprigs
- ½ cup Italian parsley, finely chopped
- ¼ tsp. of oregano, minced
- ½ tsp. of chili flakes
- 2 tbsp. of capers, drained
- 2 tbsp. of gaeta or other oil cured black olives, chopped
- 4 anchovy filets, crushed with fork

Preparation:

1. Prepare your ingredients: measure all your ingredients before you start cooking and set them on the counter.
2. Place the bass in the pesto marinade for about 30 minutes.
3. While the fish is marinating prepare the sauce.
4. Begin by searing the garlic in the olive oil.
5. Add the roma tomatoes, salt and white wine.
6. Let this simmer for about 10 minutes.
7. Now join in the rest of the ingredients.
8. While this is stewing you may begin to grill your fish.
9. Remember to clean the fish of any access oil before grilling.

Recipe Donated by **Cliff Bells** of Detroit, MI

Halibut in Herbs and Oil

Pesce a Leso con Olio e Erbette

Ingredients:

- 4 (10 oz.) slices of halibut steaks with bone in
- 3 cups salted water (2 tsp. salt in water)
- ¼ cup of white wine
- ¼ cup of extra virgin olive oil
- juice of 2 lemons
- ½ cup of finely chop italian parsley
- 2 pinches of saffron
- 2 garlic cloves, finely chopped
- 4 basil leaves, finely chopped
- 1 tsp. of dried pepperoncino or if preferred
- 2 tbsp. of pickled hot peppers, chopped

Preparation:

1. Place the fish in large tall sautéed pan with the water and wine .let the fish poach in the simmering water for 5 minutes on each side carefully take the fish out with large flat tool so it does not break and put in shallow bowl
2. Place all the herbs, raw garlic and saffron on top of fish
3. Pour the hot fish broth over the herbs
4. Squeeze the juice of 2 lemons over all ingredients
5. Pour the virgin olive oil over all
6. The fish and juices should be serve with garlic crostini
7. On each plate.

Recipe Donated by **Café Cortina** of Farmington Hills, MI

Island BBQ Ribs

Ingredients:

- vegetable oil spray
- 1 tbsp. of thyme leaves, dried
- 2 tsp. of kosher salt
- 1 tsp. of onion powder
- 1 tsp. of cayenne pepper
- 1 tsp. of ground black pepper
- ¼ tsp. of garlic powder

- ¼ tsp. of ground nutmeg
- ¼ tsp. of ground cloves
- ½ cup of water
- 2 tbsp. of extra virgin olive oil
- 3 pd. of pork spareribs (racks cut in half to fit into a gallon size zip-lock plastic bag)

Preparation:

1. Whisk together all the marinade ingredients in a bowl and place in a plastic bag with the ribs.
2. Chill for at least 1 hour, turning the bag occasionally to marinate evenly.
3. Place the rack in the center position and preheat the oven to 290°f.
4. Spray a sheet pan with vegetable oil.
5. Remove the ribs from the bag, discard the marinade, and lay the ribs meaty side up on the prepared sheet pan.
6. Cover tightly with aluminum foil and bake for about 2 hours, or until the meat is almost falling off the bone.
7. Remove from the oven and drain any liquid immediately.
8. Place the ribs meaty side down on the grill and grill for just about 5 minutes on each side until well-marked and heated through.
9. Cut into individual pieces to serve.
10. (If not grilling right away, cool and refrigerate baked ribs, covered for up to 3 days or until ready to grill.)

Mediterranean Grouper

Ingredients:

- ¾ pd. of grouper fillets
- 2 tsp. of olive oil
- 2 tbsp. of pine nuts
- 6 pitted green olives, cut in half
- ½ cup of sweet pimiento, drained & sliced
- salt and pepper (to taste)

Preparation:

1. Preheat oven to 400°f.
2. Line a baking sheet with aluminum foil.
3. Rinse the grouper and pat it dry with a paper towel, then season the grouper with salt and pepper (to taste).
4. Place the grouper on the foil wrapped baking sheet and drizzle oil on top.
5. Bake for 10 minutes.
6. Spoon pine nuts, olives, and pimiento on top of the fish.
7. Return to oven for 10 minutes.

Mediterranean Sea Bass

Pesce Branzino 'Mediterrano'

Ingredients:

- 4 sea bass filets
- ⅔ cup of extra virgin olive oil
- 2 tsp. of minced garlic
- 1 ½ cup of 'pomodoro veneziana' cafe' cortina
- 4 cups of roma tomatoes, coarsely chopped
- 2 tsp. of salt
- 2 cups of dry white wine
- ½ cup of basil, finely chopped,
- 2 basil sprigs
- 2 cups of Italian parsley, finely chopped
- ¼ tsp. of oregano, minced
- ½ tsp. of chili flakes
- 1 tbsp. of capers, drained
- 1 tbsp. of gaeta or other oil cured black olives (chopped)
- 4 anchovy filets, crushed with fork

Preparations:

1. Begin by searing the garlic in the olive oil.
2. Add the roma tomatoes, salt and white wine.
3. Let this simmer for about 10 minutes.
4. Add fish (important to allow fish to cook in sauce, keep filet's covered with sauce entire time of cooking.)
5. Now join in the rest of the ingredients and allow fish to simmer until desire temperature is reached.

Recipe Donated by **Café Cortina** of Farmington Hills, MI

Mojo Pork Roast

Ingredients:

- 1 (5 pd.) bone-in pork shoulder half
- sugar free Italian dressing
- juice from 2 limes
- 2 tbsp. of fresh cilantro, chopped
- 1 tbsp. of kosher salt
- ¼ tsp. of ground black pepper
- 3 bay leaves

Preparation:

1. Preheat oven to 325°.
2. Score the fat and skin on the pork shoulder.
3. Place the shoulder in a roasting pan lined with a rack, and pour the dressing over it.
4. Rub the remaining ingredients into the shoulder.
5. Roast uncovered for 1 hour.
6. Remove from the oven and loosely cover the shoulder with aluminum foil, like a pup tent.
7. Return to over, basting every 15 to 20 minutes, until the meat pulls from the bone easily. This should take approximately 1.5 hours.
8. Remove from heat and allow to cool for 5 minutes.
9. Trim off fat, than cut into thin slices.

Italian Dressing

Ingredients:

- 2 cups of olive oil
- ¼ cup of lemon juice
- ¼ cup of balsamic vinegar
- 1 tsp. of salt
- 1 tsp. of sugar substitute
- 1.2 tsp. of oregano, dried
- ½ tsp. of thyme, ground
- ½ tsp. of onion powder
- 2 garlic cloves, crushed

Preparation:

1. Vigorously mix all ingredients in covered container.
2. Refrigerate overnight and after use.

Moroccan Roasted Chicken

Ingredients:
- 1 whole roasted chicken
- 2 bunches of asparagus

Black Olive Butter Sauce:
- 1 cup of beef stock
- ¼ cup of black dried cured olives, pureed
- ¾ pd. of un-salted butter

Moroccan Marinade:
- 1 lemon
- ½ oz. of shallots, minced
- ½ oz. of garlic, minced
- 1 oz. of olive oil
- 2 oz. of fresh ginger, grated
- ½ tsp. of turmeric

Preparation:
1. Pre heat oven to 350 degrees.
2. For the marinade, zest the lemon and chop up fine with a knife. Blend the rest of the ingredients in a spice grinder or mortar and pestle.
3. To marinade the chicken use all of the mix and rub underneath the skin of the chicken. It is important for maximum flavor to get the marinade on the thigh and leg of the chicken. Let it marinade for a minimum of 2 hours before cooking.
4. Roast the chicken in the oven for 1 hour or until it reaches an internal temperature of 165 degrees.
5. For the sauce place the beef stock in a sauce pot and reduce by two thirds. Add the pureed olives. To finish the sauce, cube butter into ½ inch pieces. Make sure that the butter is cold. Put your beef olive reduction on low heat and slowly mix in the butter cubes. Use a whisk and keep stirring until all of the butter is incorporated. Season with salt and pepper. Keep the sauce on a warm spot on the stove to keep it from breaking.
6. Cut the root end off of the asparagus and sprinkle olive oil, salt and pepper on top. Place on a sheet tray and cook for 15 minutes.
7. When the chicken is done, let it rest for 10 minutes. If you cut it to soon all of the juices will run out and it will become dry.

Recipe Donated by **Logan - An American Restaurant**, Ann Arbor MI

Rack of Lamb

Ingredients:

- 1 rack of lamb, buy at a butcher and have them remove the fat cap
- 1 head of cauliflower
- 2 oz. of ponzu. (citrus soy sauce, found at most Asian stores)

Procedure:

1. Preheat the oven to 350 degrees.
2. Cut the cauliflower into 1 inch floweret's, coat with canola oil and spread evenly on a sheet tray and roast for 35 minutes. Half way thru the cooking process, rotate the sheet tray to allow even cooking. You will know when it is done when a nice golden brown color is achieved.
3. Season the rack of lamb and cook either by grilling or sautéing to the desired temperature that you desire.
4. To finish the cauliflower toss with the *ponzu*.

Recipe Donated by **Logan - An American Restaurant**, Ann Arbor MI

Yogurt Sauce

Ingredients:

- 8 oz. of Greek yogurt
- 1 garlic clove, diced
- ¼ oz. of shallot (diced)
- 2 sprigs of fresh mint, chiffonade

Procedure:

1. Place the garlic, shallot and yogurt into a blender and mix till a smooth texture.
2. Season with salt, pepper and the fresh mint.
3. This sauce can be made days before serving.

Recipe Donated by **Logan - An American Restaurant**, Ann Arbor MI

Sea Scallops in a Sherry Sauce

Coquille St. Jacques a la Crème aux Xeres

Ingredients:
- 4 oz. of olive oil
- 1 ¾ pd. of sea scallops
- 4 cups of mushrooms, quartered
- 1 tsp. of garlic, minced
- 2 cups of dry sherry
- 2 cups of heavy cream
- 2 tsp. of chives, chopped (to garnish)
- salt and pepper

Preparation:
1. Season the sea scallops with salt and pepper.
2. Heat large saute' pan with olive oil until smoking.
3. Carefully put scallops in pan, add mushrooms.
4. Let scallops brown on first side then flip them and turn heat down.
5. When scallops feel slightly firm, remove them and place on serving platter.
6. Continue cooking the mushrooms until tender.
7. Add garlic, stir in and saute' briefly (till aroma). Do not brown garlic.
8. Remove mushrooms and garlic with slotted spoon and place them around and on top of scallops.
9. Discard remaining oil.
10. Add sherry. Bring to a boil.
11. Reduce by half. Add cream.
12. Reduce until thickened and glossy.
13. Add salt (to taste).
14. Drain and discard the liquid that was released from the scallops and mushrooms.
15. Pour sauce over scallops and sprinkle with chives.

Recipe Donated by **The Earle** of Ann Arbor, MI

Seared Scallops with Oxtail Ragu

Ingredients:

- 8-16 large sea scallops
- 2 pd. of fresh oxtail
- 1 carrot
- 1 small sweet onion
- 1 stick of celery
- 2 tbsp. of fresh lemon zest
- 2 tbsp. of parsley, chopped
- ½ cup of red wine
- ½ cup of plum tomatoes, stewed
- 1 cup of water
- 1 bay leaf
- 1 cinnamon stick
- 1 tbsp. of *garam masala* spice blend
- salt and pepper (to taste)

Preparation:

1. In a large pot heat 1 tbsp. of oil till hot, but not smoking.
2. Season oxtails with *garam masala* and salt.
3. Sear oxtails till caramelized.
4. Dice carrot, celery, and onion. Add them to pot with the oxtails. Season with a pinch of salt and pepper.
5. Sauté till onions are translucent.
6. Add red wine to de-glaze the pot. Reduce wine by half.
7. Add water, stewed tomatoes, and bay leaf to the pot.
8. Bring to a boil, then reduce to low heat and cover tightly.
9. Cook over low heat for 3 hours, add water if needed.
10. When meat is falling off the bone, it is done. Add lemon zest and parsley to ragu. Season with salt and pepper.
11. Brush scallops with oil, and season with salt and pepper.
12. Sear in a very hot pan till caramelized on one side.
13. Turn pan off and flip scallops to just sear the bottom. Scallops should be served medium rare to medium.
14. Spoon the oxtail onto plate and arrange the seared scallops.
15. Add more lemon zest and parsley for garnish if desired.

Recipe Donated by **Cliff Bells** of Detroit, MI

Shrimp with Rosemary and Arugula

Gamberi al Rosmarino e Rucola

Ingredients:

- 20 shrimp (size 21-25, peeled and deveined)
- 2 oz. of olive oil
- 4 oz. of white wine
- 2 tsp. of garlic, minced
- 2 pinches of rosemary, chopped
- 2 pinches of red pepper, crushed
- ½ tsp. of cayenne
- salt and pepper
- ½ cup of tomatoes, diced very small
- 1 bunch of arugula, stemmed and washed

Preparation:

1. Season shrimp with salt, black pepper and cayenne.
2. Heat olive oil.
3. Sauté shrimp on medium heat till 2/3 cooked, remove from pan.
4. In remaining olive oil, sauté garlic, rosemary and crushed red pepper briefly (less than a minute).
5. Turn heat down, do not brown garlic.
6. Add white wine and tomatoes.
7. Bring to a boil.
8. Reduce until thickened.
9. Add few pinches of salt and add shrimp back in for a minute or two.
10. Serve on arugula leaves.

Recipe Donated by **The Earle** of Ann Arbor, MI

Spicy Sausage and Ground Beef Meatballs

Ingredients:

- 1 pd. of sausage
- 1 pd. of ground beef
- 3 eggs
- 2 tbsp. of onions, minced
- ½ pd. of shredded cheddar cheese
- black pepper (to taste)

Preparation:

1. Preheat oven to 350°.
2. In a large bowl, combine all ingredients and mix well.
3. Roll mixture into 1-½" balls and place on cookie sheet that has been coated with non-stick cooking spray.
4. Bake for 20 to 25 minutes.

NOTE: This will leave you with about 50 meatballs, so feel free to freeze the extra for a quick meal or snack.

Swordfish 'Tireno'

Pesce Spada 'Tireno'

Ingredients:

- ⅔ cup of extra virgin olive oil
- 2 tsp. of garlic, minced
- 3 cups of roma tomatoes, coarsely chopped
- 1 tsp. of salt
- 4 swordfish steaks (½ pd. each)
- 1 cup of dry white wine
- ½ cup of basil, finely chopped
- 2 basil sprigs
- ½ cup of Italian parsley, finely chopped
- ¼ tsp. of oregano, minced
- ½ tsp. of chili flakes
- 2 tbsp. of capers, drained
- 2 tbsp. of gaeta or other oil cured black olives, chopped
- 4 anchovy filets, crushed with fork

Preparation:

1. Prepare your ingredients: measure all your ingredients before you start cooking and set them on the counter.
2. In a 14" skillet heat ½ cup of the olive oil over medium-high heat and add the garlic.
3. Cook 30 seconds, or until the garlic barley begins to take on color (cooking the garlic longer will make it acrid)
4. Add the tomatoes to the skillet; season with salt and cook for five minutes, stirring often.
5. Add the swordfish steaks in a single layer.
6. Pour in ½ cup of the wine.
7. Cook the swordfish for five minutes on each side, turning once, for a total of ten minutes.
8. Remove the swordfish from the skillet to a tray and set aside.
9. Fold the chopped basil, parsley, oregano, chili, capers, olives and anchovies into the tomato sauce in the skillet, reduce the heat to medium-low, and cook for five minutes.
10. Add the remaining wine and return the swordfish to the skillet, still in a single layer.
11. Cook the swordfish for three minutes on each side, turning once, for a total of six more minutes.
12. The sauce should be reduced and the swordfish should be tender when poked gently with a fork.
13. Transfer the swordfish and its sauce to a serving platter and drizzle evenly with the remaining olive oil.
14. Garnish with the basil sprigs and serve hot.

Recipe Donated by **Café Cortina** of Farmington Hills, MI

Tuscan Steak with Sauce Ammoglio

Ingredients:

- 2' steak, ribeye or porterhouse
- Coarse sea salt
- Freshly cracked pepper
- Extra virgin olive oil
- Ammoglio Sauce (below)

Preparation:

1. Allow the steak to come to room temperature – usually 1 hour.
2. Season the steak well with salt and pepper.
3. Pre-heat oven to 450 degrees. Pre-heat a cast iron skillet until smoking with a little olive oil.
   Warning- turn on the exhaust fan or open the window as the steak will spit and smoke when you put it in the cast iron pan.
4. With tongs, place steak in center of the pan and cook for about 4 minutes.
5. Flip steak and place it in the oven for 5 to 6 minutes.
6. Remove from oven and allow it to rest for about 5 minutes.
7. Carve and serve with the sauce ammoglio

Recipe Donated by **Café Muse** of Royal Oak, MI

Ammoglio Sauce

- 2-3 tomatoes (seeded/roughly chopped)
- 2 garlic cloves
- ¼ cup of basil (fresh)
- 1 tbsp. of olive oil
- 1 tsp. of pepper (freshly cracked)
- ½ tsp. of salt
- 2 tbsp. of balsamic

Preparation:

1. In a small food processor pulse garlic and salt together until it is almost a liquid.
2. Add basil and peppercorns and continue to pulse.
3. Add tomatoes and pulse until desired consistency.
4. Stir in balsamic.

Recipe Donated by **Café Muse** of Royal Oak, MI

Tuscan Veal with Lemon & Mushrooms

Vitello Tosca con Funghi al Limone

Ingredients:

- 2 (8 oz.) veal cuts, chopped
- low GI baking flour
- 2 eggs
- 2 tbsp. of parsley, chopped
- ½ cup of parmesan reggiano, grated
- 1 ½ cup of porcini mushrooms, cut julienne style

- ¼ cup of olive oil
- 1 lemon, juiced
- 1 cup of white wine
- 1 ½ cup of veal stock, slightly thickened
- salt (to taste)

Preparation:

1. Start by pounding the veal chop.
2. In a medium bowl whisk together the eggs, parsley, and parmesan. This should be a slightly thick batter.
3. Place the veal chop in the flour, then in the batter.
4. Put about 1 cup of olive oil in the pan at medium plus heat.
5. Gently place the veal chop in the hot oil.
6. Let the first side sear for about 1 minute.
7. Flip the chop and place in the oven at 375 f for about 5 minutes.
8. Take the pan out and add the mushrooms to the veal.
9. Sauté for 1 minute and add the remaining ingredients.

Recipe Donated by **Café Cortina** of Farmington Hills, MI

Lunches

* ❖ BLT Lettuce Wrap
* ❖ Chicken with Rosemary & Garlic
* ❖ Ham Rolls with Cream Cheese and Chives
* ❖ Lettuce Wrap (meat of choice)
* ❖ Meatloaf
* ❖ Mediterranean Chicken Wings
* ❖ Mild Lamb Stew
* ❖ Reuben Sandwich
* ❖ Seared Tuna Sashimi
* ❖ Spicy Beef
* ❖ Spicy Chicken with Boiled Eggs
* ❖ Steak Bites

Remember, be wary with any salad dressing and check the sugar content before use. When in doubt, use as sparingly as possible... if at all!

BLT Lettuce Wrap

Ingredients:

- 4 slices of bacon
- 1 large leaf of lettuce
- ½ a sliced tomato
- Mayonnaise

Preparation:

1. Spread mayonnaise on lettuce.
2. Add bacon and tomato slices
3. Roll up the lettuce wrap and enjoy!

Chicken with Rosemary And Garlic

Pollo con Rosmarino e Aglio

Ingredients:

- 8 boneless chicken breasts, skin on
- 20 medium garlic cloves
- 4 oz. of olive oil
- ½ pd. of baby carrots, blanched till almost tender)
- 3 artichokes, trimmed down to hearts only
- 3 cups of mushrooms, quartered
- 2 ½ tbsp. of rosemary, chopped)
- salt and pepper

Preparation:

1. Using sharp knife, trim outer leaves from artichokes.
2. Continue trimming until you are down to the heart.
3. Remove fuzzy choke part and cut hearts into wedges.
4. Blanch artichoke wedges in water with a squeeze of lemon until tender.
5. Set aside to cool a bit.
6. Season chicken breasts with salt and pepper.
7. Sprinkle half the rosemary on chicken breasts.
8. Heat olive oil in large pan.
9. When smoking, add chicken breasts (skin side down).
10. Add garlic cloves and carrots.
11. Sear until golden brown.
12. Flip breasts and add artichokes and quartered mushrooms.
13. Sprinkle vegetables with remaining rosemary and a salt and black pepper.
14. Roast in 375 degree oven until done, approximately 15-20 minutes.

Recipe Donated by **The Earle** of Ann Arbor, MI

Ham Rolls with Cream Cheese and Chives

Ingredients:
- 1 package of sliced ham
- 1 package of cream cheese
- 1 tbsp. of chives

Preparation:
1. Soften the cream cheese by mixing it.
2. Chop up the chives and mix them with the cream cheese.
3. Spread onto the slices of ham.

.

Lettuce Wrap (meat of choice)

Ingredients:
- Head of lettuce (your choice of type)
- 2 slices of meat of your choice (roast beef, ham, turkey, etc.)
- 1 slice of cheese, per wrap (provolone, mozzarella, cheddar, etc.)
- Tomato slices
- Condiments of choice (use the recipes listed here or low sugar alternatives, for example: mayonnaise, mustard, etc.)

Preparation:
1. Place the slices of lunch meat and a slice of tomato on top of the leaves of lettuce.
2. Add the cheese.
3. Apply condiments as desired (in moderation).
4. Wrap up the meat, tomatoes and condiments with the leaves of lettuce.

Meatloaf

Ingredients:

- 1 ½ pd. of ground beef
- 1 cup of pork rind crumbs
- 1 egg
- ⅓ cup of tomato sauce
- 2 tbsp. of parsley
- 2 tbsp. of Italian spices
- ½ cup of parmesan, grated
- ¼ cup of onion, chopped
- ¼ cup of green pepper, chopped
- salt and pepper (to taste)

Preparation:

1. Mix all ingredients together in a bowl, making sure to distribute pork rind crumbs evenly.
2. Shape mixture into a loaf and place in a shallow nonstick baking pan.
3. Bake in a preheated oven at 350 degrees for 1 hour.

Mediterranean Chicken Wings

Ingredients:
- 2 ½ pd. of chicken wings, trimmed and separated
- 1 cup of yogurt (see below)
- 2 tbsp. of ginger
- 6 garlic cloves, minced
- 1 ½ tsp. of curry powder
- ¼ tsp. of turmeric
- ½ tsp. of cumin
- ½ tsp. of dry mustard
- 2 tsp. of red pepper flakes
- 1 lemon, juiced
- 3 tbsp. of vegetable oil
- salt and pepper (to taste)

Preparation:
1. In a large bowl, mix all ingredients.
2. Marinade wings for at least two hours at room temperature.
3. Remove the wings from the marinade and place on a broiling rack.
4. Save the marinade
5. Broil the wings for about 20 minutes, until browned and cooked through.
6. Baste wings with marinade every 10 minutes.

Yogurt

Ingredients:
- 1 quart of milk
- 1 cup of heavy cream
- 1 tbsp. of plain yogur

Preparation:
1. Mix milk and cream together and boil in a saucepan.
2. Remove from heat and allow to cool to room temperature.
3. Stir in yogurt.
4. Cover and keep in a warm place for approximately 20-30 hours.

Mild Lamb Stew

Yebg Kikil Wot

Ingredients:

- 3 pd. of lamb ribs, well cleaned and fat cut the ribs
- 10 oz. of shallots, chopped
- 4 oz. of *niter kibe* (clarified spiced butter)
- 1 tbsp. of garlic
- 1 tbsp. of ginger
- 1 tbsp. of turmeric
- salt (to taste)
- 6 cups of water
- 3 jalapeno peppers

Preparation:

1. Cut the lamb ribs to bite size and boil the meat (this will take away the mutton flavor from the meat).
2. In a deep pot, sauté the shallots.
3. Add the *niter kibe*, water, and boiled lamb to the pot, stirring to mix ingredients.
4. Mix in spices, jalapeno peppers and salt.
5. Boil for 1 hour.

Recipe Donated by **The Blue Nile** of Ferndale, MI

Reuben Sandwich

Ingredients:

- 2 slices of rye bread
- 2 slices of gruyere or Swiss cheese
- 1 cup of coleslaw
- 4 thick slices of pastrami or corned beef

- 3 tbsp. of thousand island dressing
- 1 tbsp. of butter, unsalted and softened

Preparation:

1. Spread 1 tbsp. of thousand island dressing on the first slice of rye, then a slice of cheese and half of the coleslaw. Then add all of the pastrami or corned beef.
2. Add 1 tbsp. of the thousand island dressing on top of the pastrami or corned beef, then add the remaining coleslaw and slice of cheese.
3. Spread the last tbsp. of thousand island dressing on the remaining piece of rye bread, and place it on top of the sandwich.
4. Spread the butter along the outside of the sandwich.
5. In a frying pan over medium heat, place the sandwich and press firmly with a spatula. Cook for approximately 3 to 4 minutes, or until the cheese has melted and the rye bread is crisp.
6. Flip the sandwich and repeat the process.

Seared Tuna Sashimi

Ingredients:
- 1 pd. of sushi grade tuna (can buy at any reputable fish monger)
- 2 fennel pods each
- 2 sprigs of tarragon
- 1 tab of ground coriander
- 1 bunch of baby arugula

Preparation:
1. Thinly slice the fennel, perpendicular to the grain. Stopping once you start to see the core of the vegetable.
2. Thinly slice the baby arugula and mix with the fennel. Toss with the lemon vinaigrette.
3. Season the tuna with salt on both sides of the fish.
4. Sear the fish on high heat with canola oil on one side of the fish. Let a nice golden brown crust form.
5. Pull out of the pan and liberally sprinkle with the coriander powder.
6. For presentation, put four equal portions of the fennel salad in the middle of the plate. Thinly slice the fish and place on top of the salad.

Recipe Donated by **Logan - An American Restaurant**, Ann Arbor MI

Lemon Vinaigrette

Ingredients:
- ½ oz. of lemon juice
- 2 oz. of olive oil
- ½ oz. of shallots, minced
- salt and pepper (to taste)

Preparation:
1. In a blender, mix the olive oil, lemon juice, and shallots.
2. Salt and pepper (to taste).
3. Blend till emulsified (till the ingredients combine).

Recipe Donated by **Logan - An American Restaurant**, Ann Arbor MI

Spicy Beef

Ye Siga Wot

Ingredients:

- 2 pd. of red meat cut into cubes
- 2 cups of onions, chopped
- 6 oz. of *niter kibe* (clarified spiced butter)
- 4 cups of water
- 1 tbsp. of garlic
- 1 tbsp. of ginger
- 6 tbsp. of *berbere* (Ethiopian spice mix)
- 1 tbsp. of *mekelesha* (Ethiopian spice)

Preparation:

1. In a medium size pot, cook onions, garlic, and ginger for 3 minutes with medium high heat.
2. Add *berbere* and butter, stirring frequently.
3. Cook for 15 minutes.
4. Add meat and cook for 10 minutes.
5. Add water and salt, then bring to boil with high heat, stirring frequently.
6. Reduce the heat to very low for 60 minutes.
7. Remove from the heat.

Recipe Donated by **The Blue Nile** of Ferndale, MI

Spicy Chicken with Boiled Eggs

Doro Wot

Ingredients:

- 1 whole chicken
- 4 cups of shallots, chopped
- 1 cup of *niter kibe* (clarified spiced butter)
- ½ cup of *berbere* (Ethiopian spice mix)
- 1 tbsp. of cardamom
- 1 tbsp. of garlic, diced
- 1 tbsp. of ginger, diced
- 1 tbsp. of *mekelesha* (Ethiopian spice)
- 4 cups of water
- salt (to taste)
- 6 eggs (hard boiled)

Preparation:

1. Cut chicken into four parts.
2. Remove the skin off and wash the chicken thoroughly.
3. Soak chicken in fresh lemon juice for a few hours.
4. In a medium pot, sauté the onion till brown.
5. Add garlic, ginger, butter, ½ cup of water.
6. Stir for 5 minutes.
7. Put the chicken in the pot and cook for 25 minutes.
8. Add the remaining water, stirring slowly.
9. As the sauce starts to thicken, add cardamom & hard boiled eggs.
10. Simmer for 20 minutes with low heat.

Recipe Donated by **The Blue Nile** of Ferndale, MI

Steak Bites

Ingredients:

- 1 pd. of sirloin steak or beef tips
- ½ cup of red wine
- 2 tbsp. of butter

- ½ tsp. of Italian seasoning
- 1 tsp. of garlic, minced
- salt and pepper (to taste)

Preparation:

1. Cut the meat into bite size chunks.
2. Season with the Italian seasoning.
3. In a large zip lock bag, combine ¼ a cup of red wine, garlic, and salt. Mix the ingredients well, then add the beef.
4. Marinate for overnight, flipping the bag occasionally.
5. Heat a skillet to medium high to high heat. As the pan heats, add the some of the remaining red wine, then add the butter, allowing it to melt and brown (but not blacken).
6. Place the meat in the pan in a single layer. If the meat doesn't sizzle, your pan isn't hot enough.
7. Let the meat cook for 30 to 45 seconds without interruption, then flip them over and repeat the process. The goal is to sear the outside of the meat chunks without cooking the inside.
8. Move the meat to a clean plate, and repeat steps 5 – 7 for any remaining meat.
9. Once all meat has been cooked, pour the wine/butter mixture from the skillet over the cooked steak bites.

Salads

- Blue Cheese Steak Salad
- Celery, Walnut, and Lemon Thyme Salad
- Chicken Caesar Salad
- Cocoa/Cinnamon/Chili Beef Carpaccio
- Cucumber Salad
- Duck Salad
- Ethiopian Salad
- Farro Salad with Whipped Goat Cheese
- Garden Salad (with Grilled Chicken or Steak)
- Greek Salad with Chicken
- Gruyere Cheese Caesar Salad
- Marinated Kale Salad
- Peanut Kale Salad
- Spinach Salad
- Tuna and Avocado Salad

Remember, be wary with any salad dressing and check the sugar content before use. When in doubt, use as sparingly as possible... if at all!

Blue Cheese Steak Salad

Ingredients:

- 1 pd. of skirt steak
- mixed lettuce greens
- 2 tbsp. of olive oil
- 2 cups of cherry tomatoes, halved
- ½ cup of blue cheese
- 3 tbsp. of chives, minced
- 3 tbsp. of red onions, finely chopped
- Salt and pepper to taste

Preparation:

1. Season steak with salt and pepper.
2. Heat a skillet to medium high to high heat, and then add olive oil. Cast a drop of water into the oil when you feel it is hot enough, if it snaps and crackles you may proceed.
3. Add the steak to the skillet and let it cook uninterrupted for 5 minutes. Turn and continue cooking for 3 minutes. (medium rare)
4. Remove the steak and allow it to cool for 5 minutes. Cut into strips.
5. Mix the mixed lettuce greens, cherry tomatoes, and blue cheese on a plate with the blue cheese dressing. Add the steak.
6. Sprinkle the onions and chives as garnish.

Blue Cheese Dressing

Ingredients:

- 1 cup of sour cream
- 1 cup of mayonnaise
- ½ cup of blue cheese crumbles
- 3 cloves of garlic, minced
- 2 tbsp. of green onions, finely chopped
- ½ tsp. of pepper, freshly ground
- ½ tsp. of hot sauce
- Pinch of salt

Preparation:

1. Add all ingredients in a bowl and mix thoroughly with a fork.
2. If you wish a smoother dressing, use a blender to mix.
3. Cover, and refrigerate.

Celery, Walnut, and Lemon Thyme Salad

Ingredients:
- 6 ribs celery
- 1 cup walnuts
- 6 sprigs lemon thyme leaves, stripped from stalks

Preparation:
1. Wash and slice the celery ribs diagonally.
2. In a salad bowl, toss the celery with walnuts and thyme sprigs.

Lemon Thyme Dressing

Ingredients:
- 2 tbsp. olive oil
- 2 tbsp. apple juice
- 1 tbsp. lemon juice
- 1 tbsp. fresh thyme leaves
- 1 tsp. celery seeds
- Salt and pepper to taste

Preparation:
1. Combine the oil, apple juice, lemon juice, thyme leaves, celery seeds, and a pinch each of salt and pepper in a lidded container.
2. Shake well to mix.
3. Pour over the salad.

Chicken Caesar Salad

Ingredients:

- 1 head of romaine lettuce
- 2 grilled chicken breasts
- 3 slices of bacon
- ¼ cup of parmesan, freshly grated

Preparation:

1. Grill chicken breasts, then cut into bite size chunks.
2. Cut bacon into small chunks.
3. Cut, wash and dry romaine lettuce.
4. Add Caesar dressing, parmesan, bacon, and chicken to lettuce, and mix well.

Caesar Salad Dressing

Ingredients:

- 1 garlic clove, finely chopped
- 4 tbsp. of Greek yogurt
- 3 oz. of parmesan, grated
- 1 tbsp. of olive oil
- 1 tsp. of dijon mustard
- 1 tsp. of lemon juice
- Salt and pepper to taste

Preparation:

1. Pound the garlic into a pulp, then add to a bowl.
2. Add yogurt, olive oil, garlic, parmesan, Dijon mustard, and lemon juice.
3. Whisk until items combine, and season to taste.

Cocoa/Cinnamon/Chili Beef Carpaccio

Ingredients:

- 6 oz. of black angus beef tenderloin
- ½ tsp. of cocoa powder (unsweetened)
- ½ tsp. of chili powder (dried)
- ½ tsp. of ceylon cinnamon (ground)
- Salt and pepper (to taste)

- 8 oz. of wild mushrooms (any type will work for this)
- 1 - 2 bunches of frisée or any other fresh leafy green
- 2 tbsp. of red wine vinegar
- 4 tbsp. of olive oil

Beef Preparation:

1. Start by mixing all dried spices with a pinch of salt and pepper.
2. Add 1 tbsp. of oil to this dry mix. This will form a wet rub for the beef tenderloin.
3. Rub this over the beef, make sure to coat thoroughly.
4. Heat a cast iron pan till very hot.
5. Sear the outside of the tenderloin... not the flat sides! Sear around the outside till it is charred, but be certain not to cook the tenderloin, as it is to be served very rare.
6. Set tenderloin aside to cool. If desired, it can be placed in the freezer to chill quickly.

Salad Preparation:

1. In a mixing bowl combine the vinegar and oil together.
2. Season with salt and pepper (to taste).
3. Slice mushrooms if needed.
4. Mix the frisée and mushrooms with the vinaigrette. Set aside.

Presentation:

1. Slice the chilled tenderloin carpaccio style (cut into thin ribbons, as thin as possible).
2. Lay the sliced tenderloin to cover the bottom of a plate.
3. Heap the salad mixture into the center of the tenderloin.

Recipe Donated by **Cliff Bells** of Detroit, MI

Cucumber Salad

Ingredients:
- 2 cucumbers, thinly sliced
- 4 green onions, thinly sliced
- 3 small tomatoes
- 2 tbsp. snipped parsley

Preparation:
1. Dice and combine cucumbers, onions, tomatoes and parsley.
2. Pour creamy salad dressing over salad, then toss.
3. Chill in refrigerator for approximately 1 hour before serving.

Creamy Salad Dressing

Ingredients:
- ¼ cup sour cream
- ¼ tsp. mustard
- 2 tbsp. minced dill
- 1 tbsp. vinegar
- 1 tbsp. heavy cream
- ½ tsp. salt
- ½ tsp. pepper

Preparation:
1. Combine all ingredients, mixing thoroughly.
2. Refrigerate after use.

Duck Salad

Salad de Canard

Ingredients:

- 6 cups spring greens
- 4 duck breasts, raw and skinless
- 1 each small red and green bell pepper, roasted
- 2/3 cup red onion, julienne'
- 2 bulbs garlic, roasted until tender with olive oil
- salt and pepper
- 4-6 oz. balsamic vinaigrette (recipe below)

Preparation:

1. Season duck breasts with salt and pepper.
2. Saute' in hot olive oil until desired doneness.
3. Set aside to cool. Cut tops off garlic bulbs, coat with olive oil and roast upside down in 350 degree oven until tender.
4. Remove cloves from skins while still warm.
5. Set aside to cool. Roast peppers over open gas flame, turning to char peppers evenly until charred black all over. Let cool until warm.
6. Peel peppers and cut into thin strips.
7. Slice duck breasts thinly.
8. In mixing bowl, combine duck slices, pepper strips, garlic cloves, onion and salt and black pepper.
9. Add balsamic vinaigrette and mix well. Serve on spring greens.

Balsamic Vineagrette

Ingredients:

- ½ cup balsamic vinegar
- ¾ cup extra virgin olive oil
- salt and pepper

Preparation for Balsamic Vinaigrette:

1. Pour balsamic vinegar in mixing bowl.
2. Slowly drizzle in olive oil, while whipping.
3. Season lightly with salt and pepper.

Recipe Donated by **The Earle** of Ann Arbor, MI

Ethiopian Salad

Timatim Salata

Ingredients:

- 1 head of romaine salad
- 1 stake of tomatoes
- ¼ cup of red onions

- 1 jalapeno
- 1 lemon

Preparation:

1. Wash the romaine lettuce and cut it julienne style (into long thin strips, like a shoe lace)
2. Place lettuce into a large bowl.
3. Cut the tomato, jalepeno and red onion in the same manner (julienne).
4. Remove the seeds from the jalapeno.
5. Mix the salad together, then squeeze the lemon across it all.
6. Salt & paper (to taste).
7. Serve chilled.

Recipe Donated by **The Blue Nile** of Ferndale, MI

Farro Salad with Whipped Goat Cheese

Ingredients:

- 3 cups of faro
- 5 cups of water
- 4 oz. - goat cheese
- 1ct - squash (medium)
- 1 cup of walnuts (roasted)

- 8 oz. – watercress
- ½ cups of agave
- ½ cups of apple cider vinegar
- 3/4 cups of xvoo

Preparation:

1. Poach farro in water.
2. Add 2 tbsp. of salt.
3. Bring to boil, then reduce to a simmer for 20 minutes.
4. Whip goat cheese in food processor until smooth.
5. Peel and seed squash, then dice into quarter inch cubes.
6. Toss in oil, salt and pepper.
7. Roast in oven for 20 min.
8. Mix agave and vinegar.
9. Emulsify with xvoo.
10. In sauté pan, add 1 tbsp. of oil.
11. Sauté squash.
12. Add farro and nuts and season with salt and pepper.
13. Add 1 tbsp. of agave vinaigrette.
14. Take off heat.
15. On plate spread goat cheese.
16. Build farro mixture on top.
17. Mix watercress with vinaigrette.
18. Top off salad.

Recipe Donated by **Seva Restaurant** of Detroit, MI

Garden Salad (with Grilled Chicken or Steak)

Ingredients:

- 2 heads of romaine lettuce
- 2 tomatoes
- 1 carrot, peeled & shredded
- 1 red onion, chopped
- 1 cucumber, chopped
- salt and pepper (to taste)
- parmesan cheese
- 1 lb. of flank steak OR 3 chicken breasts, skinless

Preparation:

1. Marinate the steak/chicken breasts in 3 oz. of the dressing overnight.
2. Grill the steak/chicken breasts as desired, then slice into bite size bits.
3. Wash the lettuce and let dry in a salad spinner.
4. Grate the cheese.
5. Mix the romaine lettuce with the cheese, tomatoes, carrot, red onion, and cucumbers.
6. Season with salt and pepper then add dressing to taste.
7. Add the grilled chicken or steak, then mix and serve.

Italian Dressing

Ingredients:

- 2 cups of olive oil
- ¼ cup of lemon juice
- ¼ cup of balsamic vinegar
- 1 tsp. of salt
- 1 tsp. of sugar substitute
- 1.2 tsp. of oregano, dried
- ½ tsp. of thyme, ground
- ½ tsp. of onion powder
- 2 garlic cloves, crushed

Preparation:

1. Vigorously mix all ingredients in covered container.
2. Refrigerate overnight and after use.

Greek Salad with Chicken

Ingredients:

- 2 chicken breasts
- ½ cup of lemon juice
- 1 romaine lettuce
- 1 red onion, sliced thin
- 1 green bell pepper, chopped
- 1 red bell pepper, chopped
- 2 large tomatoes, chopped
- 1 cucumber, sliced
- 1 can of pitted black olives
- 1 cup of feta cheese, crumbled

Preparation:

1. Grill the chicken breasts, dowsing the chicken in lemon juice periodically as it cooks.
2. Remove the chicken and slice into long strips.
3. In a large salad bowl, combine the romaine lettuce, tomatoes, onions, olives, bell peppers, cucumbers and feta cheese.
4. Add the greek salad dressing and toss the salad.
5. Layer the sliced chicken breast and top and serve.

Greek Salad Dressing

Ingredients:

- ½ cup of olive oil
- ¼ cup of lime juice
- 1 garlic clove, chopped
- ½ tsp. of Dijon mustard
- 1 tsp. of salt
- ½ tsp. of basil, dried
- ½ tsp. of oregano leaves, dried
- Salt and pepper to taste

Preparation:

1. Mix together thoroughly.
2. Store in refrigerator in an air tight jar.

Gruyere Cheese Caesar Salad

Ingredients:

- 1 head of romaine lettuce
- ¼ pd. of 2 year aged gruyere cheese
- ½ oz. of garlic
- 1 oz. of dijon mustard

- 1.5 oz. of lemon juice
- 3 oz. of olive oil
- ½ oz. of shallots (minced)

Preparation:

1. Cut the romaine into 1 inch pieces. Wash the lettuce and let dry in a salad spinner.
2. To make the dressing put the garlic, dijon mustard, lemon juice, olive oil and shallots into a blender and mix till emulsified (till all the items combine).
3. Grate the cheese.
4. Mix the romaine lettuce and cheese.
5. Season with salt and pepper then add the dressing.
6. Mix and serve.

Recipe Donated by **Logan - An American Restaurant**, Ann Arbor MI

Marinated Kale Salad

Ingredients:

- 2 bunches of green kale
- ⅓ cup of extra virgin olive oil
- ⅓ cup of apple cider vinegar
- 3-4 tbsp. of agave nectar, raw (to taste)
- 1-2 tsp. of sea salt (to taste)
- 1 orange, juiced

- 1 red bell pepper, seeded and diced small
- ½ cup of carrot, shaved
- 6 radishes, thinly sliced
- ½ cup of almonds, walnuts or hemp seeds (chopped) (for protein)

Preparation:

1. Whisk liquid in a large mixing bowl.
2. Add other ingredients and massage well until all ingredients are completely covered.
3. Allow mix to marinate for at least one hour on counter or refrigerator (softens kale and brings flavors together).

Recipe Donated by **The Red Pepper Deli** of Northville, MI

Peanut Kale Salad

Ingredients:

- 3/4 c peanut oil
- 3/4 c cider vinegar
- 3 c peanuts + ½ c for garnish
- 3 t agave nectar
- 1 t salt

- 1 pd. kale
- 1 red bell pepper
- ½ pd. carrots
- ½ pd. butternut squash

Preparation:

1. Chop first five ingredients in food processor until coarse and set aside.
2. Cut kale by removing center rib and slicing thinly cross-wise.
3. Slice red pepper thinly, about 1/8."
4. Quarter carrots, then slice diagonally and thinly, about 1/8."
5. Shred butternut squash.
6. Toss vegetables together and then toss thoroughly with dressing.
7. For best flavor and texture, refrigerate mixture for 2-3 hours.
8. To serve, garnish with chopped peanuts.

Recipe Donated by **Seva Restaurant** of Detroit, MI

Spinach Salad

Ingredients:

- ½ pd. of spinach
- ¼ cup of pancetta or bacon (sautéed)
- ¼ cup of gorgonzola cheese (crumbled)

- 2 eggs
- Olive oil
- Salt and pepper (to taste)

Preparation:

1. Wash greens and dry well.
2. In a large bowl toss the spinach with the vinaigrette.
3. Divide the salad between two plates and top with pancetta and gorgonzola.
4. Fry egg, sunny side up with the olive oil.
5. Season with salt and pepper and place over the salad.

Recipe Donated by **Café Muse** of Royal Oak, MI

Tuna and Avocado Salad

Ingredients:

- 2 large hard boiled eggs
- 2 tsp. hot sauce
- 1 cup avocado, mashed
- ½ cup onion (chopped)
- 1 can tuna

- 2 tbsp. mayonnaise
- 2 tbsp. pickle relish
- fresh lemon juice
- salt, (to taste)

Preparation:

1. Peel eggs and mince with dinner fork.
2. Peel avocado and squeeze on ½ lemon juice to prevent discoloration.
3. Mash avocado in with egg.
4. Drain tuna and mix into egg/avocado, adding onions, mayonnaise, relish, salt and hot sauce.
5. Stir well and serve over a bed of fresh lettuce.

Side Dishes

- ❖ Canadian Cheddar Soup
- ❖ Collard Greens
- ❖ Crab & Avocado with Tomato
- ❖ Marinara Primavera
- ❖ Snackin' Fries
- ❖ Spicy Yellow Split Peas
- ❖ Tofu and Avocado Timbale

- ❖ Watermelon Gazpacho
- ❖ White Truffle Butternut Squash Soup
- ❖ Yellow Split Peas
- ❖ Yogurt
- ❖ Zucchini Carpaccio

Remember, be wary with any salad dressing and check the sugar content before use. When in doubt, use as sparingly as possible... if at all!

Canadian Cheddar Soup

Ingredients:
- 2 tbsp. butter
- ¼ cup onion (chopped)
- ¼ cup chopped celery
- 2 tbsp. soy flour
- ¼ tsp. dry mustard
- 1 pinch nutmeg
- 1 pinch pepper
- 3 cups chicken stock
- 1 ½ cups heavy cream
- 1 cup water
- 1 ½ cups cheddar cheese, shredded
- 1 dash worcestershire sauce

Preparation:
1. Melt butter in a heavy sauce pan.
2. Cook onions and celery until tender.
3. Add flour, mustard, nutmeg and pepper.
4. Stir, cooking for 2 – 3 minutes.
5. Add chicken stock and simmer for about 20 minutes, stirring occasionally.
6. You may want to use a hand blender to puree the mixture when done.
7. Return soup to stove, adding cream and water and bring close to boiling.
8. Immediately stir in cheese and allow to melt.
   Add dashes of salt, pepper and Worcestershire sauce (to taste).

Collard Greens

Gomen Wot

Ingredients:
- 1 bundle of collard greens
- 1 tbsp. of jalapeno (chopped)
- 2 tbsp. of red onions (chopped)
- 1 tbsp. of garlic (chopped)
- 1 tbsp. of ginger
- ½ cup of olive oil

Preparation:
1. Wash the greens thoroughly.
2. Chop the greens finely and cooked it for 20 minute and strain
3. Sauté the red onions and add all ingredients
4. Mix the cooked greens with the sautéed onions and cook for 20 minutes
1. Salt (to taste)

Recipe Donated by **The Blue Nile** of Ferndale, MI

Crab & Avocado with Tomato

Ingredients:

- 1 pd. of lump crab meat
- 1 oz. of heavy cream
- ½ oz. of dijon mustard
- ½ oz. of whole grain dijon mustard
- 2 pd. of beef steak tomatoes
- 8 sprigs of thyme
- 1 oz. of olive oil
- 2 ripe avocados

Preparation:

1. Preheat non-convection oven to 300 degrees.
2. Bring a small pot of water to a boil.
3. Score the back of the tomatoes with a knife and blanch in the boiling water for 1 to 2 minutes, till the skin starts to peel away.
4. Place the blanched tomatoes in an ice bath to cool.
5. Once tomatoes are cooled, peel off the skins and remove the core.
6. Cut the tomatoes into four pieces.
7. Remove and discard the seeds and center of the tomatoes, leaving just the outside.
8. Lay tomatoes in a single layer on a sheet tray.
9. Sprinkle olive oil, salt, pepper and thyme sprigs on top of the tomatoes.
10. Place in the oven for 1 hour.
11. Remove and cool.
12. For the crab mix, open and drain the can of crab.
13. Mix the heavy cream, both dijon mustards and season with salt and pepper (to taste).
14. Once the tomatoes are cooled, cut them all into small cubes.
15. For plating, slice the avocado and season with salt.
16. Use a half of an avocado for each person. Put two tbsp. of the oven dried tomatoes on top of the seasoned avocado then put a quarter of the crab mix on top of that.

Recipe Donated by **Logan - An American Restaurant**, Ann Arbor MI

Marinara Primavera

Ingredients:

- 4-8 zucchini spiralized depending on size
- 1 ½ cups fresh baby spinach
-
- 1 ½ cups assorted raw veggies diced small (carrots, broccoli, red peppers, etc.)
- 1 tsp. sea salt

Preparation:

1. Toss all items together in a bowl and set aside.

Marinara Sauce

- 1-2 tomatoes chopped
- ½ red pepper chopped
- ½ cup sundried tomato soaked in ½ cup water for ½ hour or you may use them packed in olive oil
- 1 clove garlic minced
- 2 tbsp. oregano
- 1-3 tsp. agave (to taste)
- ½ tsp. sea salt

Preparation:

1. Drain sun-dried tomatoes and reserve water to thin sauce if desired.
2. In a food processor or blender, pulse items until as chunky or smooth as desired.
3. Drain any water that has collected in veggie bowl.
4. Add desired amount of sauce and toss.

Recipe Donated by **The Red Pepper Deli** of Northville, MI

Snackin' Fries

Ingredients:

- 1 pd. of jicama, peeled and sliced like fries
- 2 tbsp. of extra virgin olive oil
- 2 tsp. of paprika
- 1 tbsp. of onion powder
- a pinch of garlic powder
- a pinch of cayenne
- a pinch of chili powder
- add sea salt (to taste)
- a splash of lemon juice (optional)

Preparation:

1. Toss all ingredients in a bowl and enjoy.

Spicy Yellow Split Peas

Shiro Wot

Ingredients:

- 4 tbsp. of *mitin shiro* (ground, roasted, yellow split peas)
- 4 oz. of shallots (chopped)
- 3 tbsp. of olive oil
- 3 cups of water
- Salt (to taste)

Preparation:

1. Mix 4 tbsp. of *mitin shiro* with water.
2. Mix vigorously to dissolve lumps.
3. Cook shallots and olive oil in a small pot for 4 minutes.
4. Add water and bring to boil.
5. Pour *mitin shiro* mixture into pot.
6. Stir continuously.
7. Let simmer for 40 minutes over low heat until sauce is thick and smooth.

Recipe Donated by **The Blue Nile** of Ferndale, MI

Tofu and Avocado Timbale

Ingredients:

- 8 oz. of tofu
- 2 avocados
- 2 ripe heirloom tomatoes
- Fresh cilantro
- 3 tbsp. of lime juice

- 6 tbsp. of extra virgin olive oil
- 4 pieces of thinly sliced pumpernickel bread (toasted till crisp)
- Salt and pepper (to taste)

Preparation:

1. Start by cutting all tofu, avocado, and tomatoes into cubes of relative size.
2. Mince cilantro.
3. Combine all ingredients in bowl.
4. Add lime juice and olive oil.
5. Season with salt and pepper (to taste).
6. Add minced cilantro.
7. Gently mix ingredients together.
8. Serve with pumpernickel crisps.

Recipe Donated by **Cliff Bells** of Detroit, MI

Watermelon Gazpacho

Ingredients:

- 4 cups of watermelon, seeded and pureed
- 1 cup of watermelon, seeded and diced small
- 1 cup peeled, seeded cucumber diced sm
- 1 cup of seeded tomatoes (diced) small
- ¼ cup of green bell pepper (diced) small
- ¼ cup of red bell pepper (diced) small
- 2 tbsp. of sweet or green onion, minced
- 1 tsp. of ginger, minced
- 1 ½ tsp. of sea salt
- 1 lime, juiced
- ½ to 1 jalapeno, seeded and minced (depending on preferred hotness).

Preparation:

1. Puree watermelon in a blender, then place in a bowl.
2. Add remaining ingredients.
3. Chill until ready to serve.

Recipe Donated by **The Red Pepper Deli** of Northville, MI

White Truffle Butternut Squash Soup

Ingredients:

- 2 large butternut squash
- 1 quart of chicken stock
- 1 oz. of butter

- 1 medium sized onion
- 2 cloves of garlic
- 1 tab of white truffle oil

Preparation:

1. Preheat oven to 350 degrees.
2. Cut butternut squash in half and scoop out all the seeds.
3. Place on a sheet tray with parchment paper and roast for 1 hour.
4. Once the squash has cooled long enough to handle, puree in a food processor or blender. Use some of the chicken stock to let it form into a puree.
5. Mince the onion and garlic.
6. In a large soup pot melt the butter and cook the onion and garlic under low heat till they are translucent.
7. Add the squash puree and the rest of the chicken stock.
8. Bring to a simmer and cook for 30 minutes.
9. Season with salt, pepper and the truffle oil.
10. Serve with a dollop of sour cream and fresh chives.

Recipe Donated by **Logan - An American Restaurant**, Ann Arbor MI

Yellow Split Peas

Yekik Alicha Wot

Ingredients:

- 3 cups of yellow split peas
- 2 cups of red onions (chopped)
- 2 cups of olive oil
- 5 cups of water
- 1 tbsp. of ginger
- 1 tbsp. of garlic
- 1 tbsp. of turmeric
- ½ cup of white wine or honey wine
- 1 jalapeno

Preparation:

1. Wash the yellow split peas till the water is clear (this helps to remove the starch).
2. Remove the seeds from the jalapeno.
3. Cook onions in the olive oil, adding the turmeric, ginger, and garlic.
4. When the onions become translucent, add the jalapeno, yellow split peas, and water.
5. Boil 15 minute.
6. Salt (to taste)

Recipe Donated by **The Blue Nile** of Ferndale, MI

Yogurt

Ingredients:

- 1 quart milk
- 1 cup heavy cream
- 1 tbsp. plain yogurt

Preparation:

1. Mix milk and cream together and boil in a saucepan.
2. Remove from heat and allow to cool to room temperature.
3. Stir in yogurt.
4. Cover and keep in a warm place for approximately 20-30 hours.

Zucchini Carpaccio

Ingredients:

- 3 zucchini
- ¼ pd. of parmesan reggianio cheese
- 1 bunch of chives
- ½ oz. of lemon juice
- 2 oz. of olive oil
- ½ oz. of shallots (minced)

Preparation:

1. Wash and dry the zucchini.
2. Slice zucchini into very thin 1" strips. Place in bowl.
3. Grate the parmesan cheese on the small side of the cheese grater.
4. Make a lemon vinaigrette in a blender with olive oil, lemon juice, and shallots. Salt and pepper (to taste). Blend till emulsified.
5. Slice the chives.
6. Mix the zucchini, chives, and parmesan.
7. Toss with the lemon vinaigrette and season with salt and pepper.
8. Eat soon after the salad is tossed with the vinaigrette.

Recipe Donated by **Logan - An American Restaurant**, Ann Arbor MI

Breakfasts

- ❖ Bacon and Eggs
- ❖ Baked Eggs and Bacon
- ❖ Breakfast Burrito
- ❖ Faux French Toast
- ❖ Ham and Cheese Breakfast Muffins
- ❖ Oatmeal Pancakes with Yogurt & Fruit
- ❖ Scrambled Eggs with Gruyere & Salmon
- ❖ Spinach and Cheese Omelet
- ❖ Strawberry Crepes

In general, most omelets and eggs are safe on the GI scale. Just watch the additional ingredients beyond the eggs, vegetables, and cheese.

If you wish to add a slice of toast, remember to choose from the varieties that have a low to medium GI and GL. For example, pumpernickel, rye, and sourdough all have median GI and GL levels.

Bacon and Eggs

Ingredients:

- 4 egg whites (½ cup)
- 1 slice of turkey bacon
- ½ cup baby spinach leaves
- ¼ cup grated reduced-fat cheddar
- fat-free cooking spray
- 2 tbsp. flavored salsa (optional)

Preparation:

1. In a skillet coated with fat free cooking spray, scramble 4 egg whites.
2. Chop turkey bacon and stir in.
3. Add spinach leaves.
4. When spinach wilts, melt cheese on egg scramble.
5. Add zip to this dish by stirring in flavored salsa.

Baked Eggs and Bacon

Ingredients:

- 6 slices of bacon
- 6 eggs
- 1 non stick muffin pan

Preparation:

1. For each muffin cup, take one slice of bacon and wrap around 4 fingers to shape it into a circle.
2. Place in muffin cup.
3. Crack egg into the center.
4. Repeat for each serving.
5. Place muffin pan in oven and bake at 350 for about 40 minutes.

Breakfast Burrito

Ingredients:

- ¼ cup mushrooms
- ¼ cup zucchini
- ⅓ cup tomato
- 1 clove garlic
- 2 eggs
- dash cayenne pepper
- dash chili powder
- 2 tbsp. salsa
- 2 low carb tortilla shells
- mexican cheese blend

Preparation:

1. Finely chop the garlic and dice the tomato, zucchini and mushrooms.
2. Pour mixture into eggs and add the pepper and chili powder.
3. Stir until blended.
4. Add mixture to skillet and scramble until done.
5. Place a serving in one low carb tortilla shell, sprinkle with cheese and salsa.

Faux French Toast

Ingredients:

- 2 eggs
- ¼ cup of heavy whipping cream
- 2 packages of sugar substitute
- cinnamon (to taste)
- ½ of a 3 oz. bag of unflavored pork rinds

Preparation:

1. Crush the pork rinds as finely as you can without turning them into a powder.
2. Mix together the eggs, cream, sweetener and cinnamon and pour into bowl with pork rinds.
3. Stir and allow mixture to soak until you have a thick, goopy batter.
4. Pour in batter and fry "pancake style" in butter, browning both sides until done.
5. Serve with your favorite low carb syrup.

Ham and Cheese Breakfast Muffins

Ingredients:

- 6 large eggs, separated
- 1 tsp. cream of tartar
- ½ cup cottage cheese
- ¼ cup dr. atkins bake mix
- 1 tsp. salt
- 2 tbsp. green onion, minced

- 2 tbsp. butter, melted
- 1 tsp. sugar twin sugar substitute
- 2 cups ham
- 1 cup cheddar cheese, cubed
- ½ cup cream

Preparation:

1. Place separated egg whites into a mixing bowl along with the cream of tartar and set aside.
2. Place egg yolks in another bowl and add remaining ingredients one by one, making sure to stir after each addition.
3. Whip egg whites and cream of tartar until still, then fold into egg yolk mixture.
4. Pour mixture evenly into nonstick, buttered muffin pans.
5. Bake at 350 degrees for 30 – 35 minutes.

Oatmeal Pancakes with Yogurt & Fruit

Ingredients:

- 2 cups of quick oats
- 4 egg whites
- ½ tsp. of vanilla
- ½ tsp. of cinnamon

- ½ tsp. of baking powder
- ¼ cup of pumpkin puree
- ½ cup of fat free milk or butter milk

Preparation:

1. Combine all ingredients.
2. Pan fry with butter or olive oil

Top with:

1. 1 cup of fat free vanilla yogurt
2. 1 cup of diced strawberries

Recipe Donated by **Café Muse** of Royal Oak, MI

Scrambled Eggs with Gruyere & Salmon

Ingredients:

- 6 whole eggs
- 1 tbsp. of half and half or water
- sea salt and fresh ground pepper (to taste)
- butter or olive oil for pan
- ¼ cup of gruyere or swiss cheese (shredded)
- 4 oz. smoked salmon (diced)
- 1 tsp. chives (minced)
- optional: asparagus

Preparation:

1. In a bowl, add the eggs, water (or half and half), & salt and pepper.
2. Whip with a fork.
3. In a non-stick sauté pan over medium heat, melt your butter and pour egg mixture in.
4. With a rubber spatula, push the eggs towards the center as they cook.
5. When the eggs are about ½ way cooked, add the cheese, salmon and chives.
6. Continue to cook until they reach the desired doneness. Café Muse suggests them a little soft.
7. Optionally, serve with freshly sautéed asparagus.

Recipe Donated by **Café Muse** of Royal Oak, MI

Spinach and Cheese Omelet

Ingredients:

- 4 eggs
- salt
- cayenne pepper
- ¼ shredded sharp cheddar cheese
- 1 tbsp. fresh chives, flat-leaf parsley or chervil
- 2/3 cup red pepper relish (see recipe)
- non stick cooking spray

Preparation:

1. Light coat an eight inch nonstick skillet with cooking spray and heat over medium high heat.
2. In a mixing bowl, beat together the eggs, one dash of salt and one dash of cayenne pepper until mixture is frothy.
3. Pour into skillet.
4. Allow the egg to set, making sure to lift the edges frequently and allow uncooked portion to run under the cooked portion.
5. Continue until egg appears glossy and cooked, but still moist.
6. Add ¾ of the cup of spinach and 2 tbsp. of red pepper relish, topping with cheese and chives.
7. Use spatula to lift up the edges of the omelet and fold in half.
8. Sprinkle with remaining spinach and red pepper relish.
9. Add additional cheese and chives (to taste).

Red Pepper Relish

Ingredients:

- 2/3 cup sweet red pepper
- 2 tbsp. chopped onion
- 1 tbsp. cider vinegar
- ¼ tsp. black pepper

Preparation:

1. Combine all ingredients in a bowl and set aside while preparing omelet. This should make about 2/3 cup of red pepper relish.

Strawberry Crepes

Ingredients:

- butter (enough to fry crepes)
- 3 large eggs
- 2/3 cup heavy cream
- 3 tbsp. dr. atkins bake mix
- 4 tbsp. sugar substitute
- 1/8 tsp. almond extract
- ¼ tsp. vanilla extract
- ½ tsp. orange zest grated

Strawberry Filling:

- 2 cups strawberries, washed, hulled and sliced
- 6 tbsp. sugar twin sugar substitute

Preparation:

1. Prepare a heavy, 8 inch skillet or crepe pan with heated butter.
2. Whisk all crepe ingredients together in mixing bowl.
3. Once the butter stops foaming, pour 1/6 crepe mixture into skillet, making sure to cover the bottom evenly.
4. Cook until bottom is browned and top is set.
5. Use a spatula to flip the crepe and brown the other side.
6. Once done, transfer to a paper towel.
7. Repeat this procedure with remaining batter and butter.
8. Next, make your filling by combining strawberries with sugar substitute.
9. Spoon about ¼ of mixture on each crepe.
10. Add light whipped cream (to taste) and garnish with remaining strawberries.

Smoothies

- ❖ Blueberry Banana Bonanza
- ❖ Chocoholics Smoothie
- ❖ Chocolate and Peanut Butter Smoothie
- ❖ Coco Banana Smoothie
- ❖ Dr. Feelgood
- ❖ Emerald Isle Smoothie
- ❖ Mango Pineapple Chill
- ❖ Mean and Green Meal In A Cup
- ❖ Peaches and Cream
- ❖ Pear and Strawberry Chiller
- ❖ Pumpkin Patch
- ❖ Strawberry Banana Delight
- ❖ Strawberry Lemonade
- ❖ Very Berry

Smoothies make a great snack or meal, feel free to experiment and make up your own varieties with low GI items.

You may also add protein powder to these mixes for a more protein rich diet. We suggest vanilla varieties.

Blueberry Banana Bonanza

Ingredients:

- 1 banana, frozen
- A handful of blueberries, frozen
- medium scoop of ice
- 16 oz. of apple juice, unsweetened
- *OPTIONAL:* 1-2 tsp. of sugar substitute (stevia or other alternative sweetener)

Preparation:

1. Combine and blend to desired consistency.

Chocoholics Smoothie

Ingredients:

- 6 oz. of yogurt, sugar free
- 8 oz. of milk
- 2 tbsp. of chocolate syrup, sugar free
- large scoop of ice
- *OPTIONAL:* 1-2 tsp. of sugar substitute (stevia or other alternative sweetener)

Preparation:

1. Combine and blend to desired consistency.

Chocolate and Peanut Butter Smoothie

Ingredients:

- 6 oz. of yogurt, sugar free
- 8 oz. of milk
- 2 tbsp. of chocolate syrup, sugar free
- 2 tbsp. of peanut butter
- large scoop of ice
- *OPTIONAL:* 1-2 tsp. of sugar substitute (stevia or other alternative sweetener)

Preparation:

1. Combine and blend to desired consistency.

Coco Banana Smoothie

Ingredients:

- 3/4 cup coconut milk
- 1 large ripe banana
- 1 tbsp. raw cacao
- large scoop of ice
- OPTIONAL: 1-2 tsp. of sugar substitute (stevia or other alternative sweetener)

- OPTIONAL: add ½ cup or raspberries or strawberries
- OPTIONAL: for extra protein and creaminess, add 1 tbsp. of nut butter (almond, cashew, or peanut butter)

Preparation:
1. Combine and blend to desired consistency.

Dr. Feelgood

Ingredients:

- 1 avocado
- ½ cup of kale
- ½ cup of spinach
- 1 celery stalk, sliced

- 1 apple, cored and sliced
- OPTIONAL: 1-2 tsp. of sugar substitute (stevia or other alternative sweetener)

Preparation:
1. Combine and blend to desired consistency.

Recipe Donated by **Seva Restaurant** of Detroit, MI

Emerald Isle Smoothie

Ingredients:

- ½ cup of orange juice
- ⅔ cup of mango
- 1 large handful of spinach
- 1 banana
- a few ice cubes to keep it cool

- 1 serving of desired green superfood
- OPTIONAL: 1-2 tsp. of sugar substitute (stevia or other alternative sweetener)

Preparation:
1. Combine and blend to desired consistency.

Mango Pineapple Chill

Ingredients:

- 1 mango, chopped
- ½ can of pineapple, unsweetened
- 12 oz. of pineapple juice, unsweetened

- *OPTIONAL:* 1-2 tsp. of sugar substitute (stevia or other alternative sweetener)

Preparation:

1. Combine and blend to desired consistency.

Mean and Green Meal In A Cup

Ingredients:

- ½ cup of lemon juice
- 1 pear or apple, cored & chopped
- 1 banana, frozen
- 1 celery stalk, chopped small
- 1 large leaf kale, chopped small

- 1 handful of fresh baby spinach
- ½ cup of ice
- 3 leaves dandelion (optional)
- *OPTIONAL:* 1 serving of green super food of choice

Preparation:

1. Combine and blend to desired consistency. If too thick to blend, add a little water.

Recipes Donated by **The Red Pepper Deli** of Northville, MI

Peaches and Cream

Ingredients:

- 2 peaches, pitted and sliced
- 6 oz. of yogurt, sugar free
- 12 oz. of milk
- 1 banana, frozen

- a few ice cubes to keep it cool
- *OPTIONAL:* 1-2 tsp. of sugar substitute (stevia or other alternative sweetener)

Preparation:

1. Combine and blend to desired consistency.

Pear and Strawberry Chiller

Ingredients:

- 1 pear, cored and sliced
- 3 large strawberries, hulled
- 1 cup of yogurt, sugar free
- ¼ cup of milk
- ½ cup of ice
- OPTIONAL: 1-2 tsp. of sugar substitute (stevia or other alternative sweetener)

Preparation:
1. Combine and blend to desired consistency.

Pumpkin Patch

Ingredients:

- 1 cup of almond milk
- ½ cup of pumpkin puree
- ½ cup of cool whip, sugar free
- ¼ tsp. of cinnamon
- ¼ tsp. of nutmeg
- a few ice cubes to keep it cool
- OPTIONAL: 1-2 tsp. of sugar substitute (stevia or other alternative sweetener)

Preparation:
1. Combine and blend to desired consistency.

Strawberry Banana Delight

Ingredients:

- 1 banana, frozen
- 1 cup of strawberries, frozen
- 6 oz. of yogurt, sugar free
- a few ice cubes to keep it cool
- OPTIONAL: 1-2 tsp. of sugar substitute (stevia or other alternative sweetener)

Preparation:
1. Combine and blend to desired consistency.

Strawberry Lemonade

Ingredients:

- 1 cup of strawberries, frozen
- 16 oz. of lemonade, sugar free
- 1 banana, frozen
- a few ice cubes to keep it cool

- *OPTIONAL:* 1-2 tsp. of sugar substitute (stevia or other alternative sweetener)

Preparation:

1. Combine and blend to desired consistency.

Very Berry

Ingredients:

- 1 banana, frozen
- ½ cup of blackberries, frozen
- ½ cup of raspberries, frozen
- ½ cup of strawberries, frozen
- ½ cup of milk

- a few ice cubes to keep it cool
- *OPTIONAL:* 1-2 tsp. of sugar substitute (stevia or other alternative sweetener)

Preparation:

1. Combine and blend to desired consistency.

Condiments, Sauces and Dressings

- Agave Ketchup
- Ammoglio Sauce
- Barbeque Sauce
- Balsamic Vinaigrette
- Balsamic Vinaigrette Dressing
- Blue Cheese Dressing
- Caesar Salad Dressing
- Guacamole
- Italian Dressing
- Ketchup
- Lemon Thyme Dressing
- Lemon Vinaigrette
- Marinara Sauce
- Pickle Relish
- Red Pepper Relish
- Thousand Island Dressing
- Yogurt Sauce

Here are a few alternative recipes for condiments and salad dressings.

Agave Ketchup

Ingredients:
- 1 ½ cups of tomato (diced)
- 1 ½ tbsp. of agave nectar, raw
- 3 tbsp. of extra virgin olive oil
- 1 tsp. of sea salt
- 1 tbsp. of apple cider vinegar
- ½ cup of sun-dried tomatoes, soaked or packed in olive oil

Preparation:
1. Drain sun-dried tomatoes and reserve soak water.
2. Blend all ingredients until smooth, using a little soak water if needed. You may use a blender or food processor.

Recipe Donated by **The Red Pepper Deli** of Northville, MI

Ammoglio Sauce

- 2-3 tomatoes (seeded/roughly chopped)
- 2 garlic cloves
- ¼ cup of basil (fresh)
- 1 tbsp. of olive oil
- 1 tsp. of pepper (freshly cracked)
- ½ tsp. of salt
- 2 tbsp. of balsamic

Preparation:
1. In a small food processor pulse garlic and salt together until it is almost a liquid.
2. Add basil and peppercorns and continue to pulse.
3. Add tomatoes and pulse until desired consistency.
4. Stir in balsamic.

Recipe Donated by **Café Muse** of Royal Oak, MI

Balsamic Vinaigrette

Ingredients:
- ½ cup balsamic vinegar
- ¾ cup extra virgin olive oil
- salt and pepper

Preparation for Balsamic Vinaigrette:
1. Pour balsamic vinegar in mixing bowl.
2. Slowly drizzle in olive oil, while whipping.
3. Season lightly with salt and pepper.

Recipe Donated by **The Earle** of Ann Arbor, MI

Balsamic Vinaigrette Dressing

Ingredients:
- 1 cup of extra virgin olive oil
- ⅓ cup of balsamic vinegar
- 1 tsp. of wholegrain mustard
- Sea salt and freshly cracked pepper (to taste)
- Immersion blender

Preparation:
1. In a cup large enough to fit the head of the blender, place the vinegar, honey, mustard and ½ tsp. salt.
2. Pulse a few times to dissolve the salt and combine the ingredients.
3. With the blender running, slowly pour in the olive oil.
4. Once all the oil is added, continue to run the blender for another 30 seconds.
5. Taste and add salt and pepper.

Recipe Donated by **Café Muse** of Royal Oak, MI

Barbeque Sauce

Ingredients:
- 1 cup of tomato paste
- 3 tbsp. of cider vinegar
- 1 tsp. of worcestershire sauce
- 1 tbsp. of garlic powder
- ½ tbsp. of onion powder
- ½ tsp. of red pepper, ground
- ½ tsp. of sugar substitute (stevia or sugar alternative)
- 1 dash of cinnamon
- 1 dash of paprika

Preparation:
1. Mix the tomato paste, cider vinegar, worchestershire sauce, garlic powder, onion powder, and red pepper in a saucepan. Bring to a boil.
2. Add in sugar substitute, mix and allow to simmer for 15 minutes.
3. Remove from heat and add cinnamon and paprika, mix and allow to cool.
4. Cover, and refrigerate.

Note: This sauce will only keep for about a week, so make as needed.

Blue Cheese Dressing

Ingredients:
- 1 cup of sour cream
- 1 cup of mayonnaise
- ½ cup of blue cheese crumbles
- 3 cloves of garlic, minced
- 2 tbsp. of green onions, finely chopped
- ½ tsp. of pepper, freshly ground
- ½ tsp. of hot sauce
- Pinch of salt

Preparation:
1. Add all ingredients in a bowl and mix thoroughly.
2. If you wish a smoother dressing, use a blender instead of a fork to mix.
3. Cover, and refrigerate.

Caesar Salad Dressing

Ingredients:
- 1 garlic clove, finely chopped
- 4 tbsp. of greek yogurt
- 3 oz. of parmesan, grated
- 1 tbsp. of olive oil
- 1 tsp. of dijon mustard
- 1 tsp. of lemon juice
- Salt and pepper to taste

Preparation:
1. Pound the garlic into a pulp, then add to a bowl.
2. Add yogurt, olive oil, garlic, parmesan, Dijon mustard, and lemon juice.
3. Whisk until items combine, and season to taste.

Creamy Salad Dressing

Ingredients:
- ¼ cup sour cream
- ¼ tsp. mustard
- 2 tbsp. minced dill
- 1 tbsp. vinegar
- 1 tbsp. heavy cream
- ½ tsp. salt
- ½ tsp. pepper

Preparation:
1. Combine all ingredients, mixing thoroughly.
2. Refrigerate after use.

Guacamole

Ingredients:
- 3 ripe avocados
- 3t lemon juice
- 1t lime juice
- 1 small red onion
- 2 small tomatoes, such as roma
- 1 small jalapeno, seeded and miced
- 2 minced garlic cloves
- 1t salt
- garnish: ¼ cup chopped cilantro

Preparation:
1. Remove the stems from the avocados, cut in half, rotating knife around the seed.
2. Discard the seed.
3. Scoop out pulp with spoon into large bowl.
4. Mash with fork, leaving some chunks for texture.
5. Finely dice tomato and onion and add to mashed avocados.
6. Add all other ingredients and gently stir, adjusting (to taste).
7. Garnish with cilantro (if desired) and serve.

Recipe Donated by **Seva Restaurant** of Detroit, MI

Italian Dressing

Ingredients:
- 2 cups of olive oil
- ¼ cup of lemon juice
- ¼ cup of balsamic vinegar
- 1 tsp. of salt
- 1 tsp. of sugar substitute
- 1.2 tsp. of oregano, dried
- ½ tsp. of thyme, ground
- ½ tsp. of onion powder
- 2 garlic cloves, crushed

Preparation:
1. Vigorously mix all ingredients in covered container.
2. Refrigerate overnight and after use.

Ketchup

Ingredients:

- 1 can of tomato paste
- 1 garlic clove, chopped
- 2 tbsp. of vinegar (preferably apple cider vinegar, but others will do)
- 1 tsp. of cloves, ground
- 1 tsp. of cinnamon
- ¾ tsp. of freshly ground pepper
- ½ tsp. of celery
- ¼ cup of water
- 8 tsp. of artificial sweetener (stevia or sugar alternatives)

Preparation:

1. Mix all items except the sweetener in a saucepan.
2. Bring to a boil, then allow to simmer for approximately 30 minutes.
3. Remove from heat and add sweetener.

Note: This sauce will only keep for about a week, so make as needed.

Lemon Thyme Dressing

Ingredients:

- 2 tbsp. olive oil
- 2 tbsp. apple juice
- 1 tbsp. lemon juice
- 1 tbsp. fresh thyme leaves
- 1 tsp. celery seeds
- Salt and pepper to taste

Preparation:

1. Combine the oil, apple juice, lemon juice, thyme leaves, celery seeds, and a pinch each of salt and pepper in a lidded container.
2. Shake well to mix.

Lemon Vinaigrette

Ingredients:

- ½ oz. of lemon juice
- 2 oz. of olive oil
- ½ oz. of shallots, minced
- salt and pepper (to taste)

Preparation:

1. In a blender, mix the olive oil, lemon juice, and shallots.
2. Salt and pepper (to taste).
3. Blend till emulsified (till the ingredients combine).

Recipe Donated by **Logan - An American Restaurant**, Ann Arbor MI

Marinara Sauce

- 1-2 tomatoes chopped
- ½ red pepper chopped
- ½ cup sundried tomato soaked in ½ cup water for ½ hour or you may use them packed in olive oil
- 1 clove garlic minced
- 2 tbsp. oregano
- 1-3 tsp. agave (to taste)
- ½ tsp. sea salt

Preparation:

1. Drain sun-dried tomatoes and reserve water to thin sauce if desired.
2. In a food processor or blender, pulse items until as chunky or smooth as desired.
3. Drain any water that has collected in veggie bowl.
4. Add desired amount of sauce and toss.

Recipe Donated by **The Red Pepper Deli** of Northville, MI

Pickle Relish

Ingredients:

- 1 jar of dill pickle spears
- 1 cup of onions, chopped
- ¼ of a red bell pepper, seeded and chopped
- ¼ of a green bell pepper, seeded and chopped
- ½ cup of sugar substitute (stevia or sugar alternatives)
- ½ tsp. of celery seed
- ½ tsp. of mustard seeds
- 2 tbsp. of cider vinegar

Preparation:

1. Drain the pickles into a non-reactive bowl and store overnight.
2. Either hand chop or use a food processor to cut the pickles, onions and peppers into the desired consistency for your relish.
3. Place vegetables in a jar and refrigerate overnight.
4. Drain liquid from vegetables into the same non-reactive bowl you placed the pickle brine, then add the celery/mustard seed and sugar substitute.
5. Add the cider vinegar to the mixed vegetables in jar.
6. Bring the brine in non-reactive bowl to a simmer for 20 to 30 minutes.
7. Pour brine back into the jar with the mixed vegetables.
8. Store in refrigerator.

Red Pepper Relish

Ingredients:

- 2/3 cup sweet red pepper
- 2 tbsp. chopped onion
- 1 tbsp. cider vinegar
- ¼ tsp. black pepper

Preparation:

1. Combine all ingredients in a bowl.
2. Cover and refrigerate.

Thousand Island Dressing

Ingredients:
- ¼ cup of mayonnaise (fat free, if preferred)
- ¼ cup of sour cream
- ¼ cup of ketchup (sugar free)
- 3 tbsp. of pickle relish (sugar free)
- 1 tbsp. of mustard

Preparation:
1. Mix the ingredients together and alter to your personal taste.
2. If you desire a sweeter blend, add in stevia or a sugar alternative.

Yogurt Sauce

Ingredients:
- 8 oz. of greek yogurt
- 1 clove of garlic (diced)
- ¼ oz. of shallot (diced)
- 2 sprigs of fresh mint, chiffonade

Procedure:
1. Place the garlic, shallot and yogurt into a blender and mix till a smooth texture.
2. Season with salt, pepper and the fresh mint.
3. This sauce can be made days before serving.

Recipe Donated by **Logan - An American Restaurant**, Ann Arbor MI

Snacks

- ❖ Applesauce
- ❖ Cheese
- ❖ Cottage Cheese
- ❖ Eaggs
- ❖ Fruit
- ❖ Meats

- ❖ Nuts
- ❖ Popcorn
- ❖ Pork Rinds
- ❖ Raw Vegetables
- ❖ Yogurt

Snack time is actually quite easy on the Patino Diet, as most fruits, vegetables, meat, and cheese are low glycemic.

When it comes to prepared foods, such as jerky and pepperoni, make sure to check over the nutritional information for sugar content.

Applesauce

Make sure to select the natural, unsweetened varieties. As always, check the labels for their sugar content! If desired, mix with cinnamon and/or artificial sweeteners.

Cheese

Feel free to enjoy cheese in all it's wonderful variety, but keep your portions moderate. You may select slices or cheese sticks, mixed with vegies or meat, or just on its own.

If you are a chip lover, look into Aged parmesan Cheese Crisps at your local health food store.

Cottage Cheese

Mix with fruit or cinnamon, if desired.

Eggs

Hard boiled eggs are a convenient snack that can be easily transported, but deviled eggs are fine as well.

Fruit

When it comes to fruit, a good rule of thumb is to choose fruits that you eat with the skin on. You can add peanut butter, nut butter, or cheese with these items.

- Strawberries
- Blueberries
- Blackberries
- Bananas
- Apples
- Pears
- Pear Apples
- Oranges
- Plums
- Peaches

Meats

Pepperoni, Sausages, Kielbasas, Lunch Meats, Beef Jerky, and similar products. If desired, these can be mixed with cheese, cream cheese, tuna salad, egg salad, or other sugar free toppings/fillings.

Lunch meats can also be a delicious snack. Just roll them up with cheese, cream cheese, tuna salad, egg salad, or other sugar free fillings.

For something a little different, nuke sliced pepperoni in the microwave for 30 seconds to create "Pepperoni Chips".

Nuts

Almonds, pistachios, peanuts, walnuts, hazelnuts, pumpkin seeds, sunflower seeds, or any other type of whole nut.

Popcorn

Avoid the microwave varieties and stick with air popped popcorn.

Pork Rinds

A delicious snack right out of the bag.

Raw Vegetables

If desired, you can eat these vegetables with peanut butter, cream cheese, hummus, yogurt dip, salsa, tuna salad, or guacamole.

- Cucumbers
- Broccoli
- Cauliflower
- Pea Pods
- Celery
- Carrots
- Peppers
- Similar Vegetables

Yogurt

Mix with fruit, nuts, or peanut butter, as desired.

Desserts

- ❖ Cookies
- ❖ Dark Chocolate
- ❖ Frozen Fruit
- ❖ Fruit
- ❖ Fudge
- ❖ Ice Cream
- ❖ Jello, Mousse & Pudding
- ❖ Specialty Desserts

WARNING!

There a number of low carb and sugar free desserts available at your local grocery store, but these items should be taken in careful moderation. Most of these items are made with artificial sweeteners, and taking these items in excess can create some uncomfortable gastric side effects.

Cookies

Sugar free and low carb varieties can be found at most local grocery stores. We recommend the peanut butter varieties for pure tastiness!

Dark Chocolate

A delicious treat, feel free to mix with peanut butter.

Frozen Fruit

Berries, Bananas and Grapes can all be frozen and eaten as a healthy frozen snack. There are also several varieties of frozen fruit bars available at your local grocer, but be careful to check the nutritional information!

Fruit

Mixed fruit makes a wonderful sweet ending to a meal. Check the snack section for our recommendations on fruit varieties.

Fudge

There are several sugar free and low carb varieties of fudge available.

Ice Cream

Again, there are several low carb and sugar free varieties available. Be careful of "no sugar added" labels, as this is NOT the same as sugar free.

My personal favorite is a Peanut Butter Pecan Sunday. Mix 1 scoop of low carb butter pecan ice cream, 2 tbsp. of peanut butter, and 2 sugar free peanut butter cookies in a bowl... and enjoy!

Jello, Mousse, and Pudding

Add light whipped cream as desired.

Specialty Desserts

There are a large number of low carb and sugar free desserts available at your local grocery store, but be warned that their advertising can be very misleading. Always check the nutritional labels for the actual sugar content and serving size.

Contributors

We have been lucky enough to have the help of several restaurants throughout the Greater Detroit area in the development of this book. These establishments offered recipes from their culinary arsenal to assist us in the development of your health regiment. We have included some information on each restaurant, as well as the recipes that they have donated, in the following section.

The Blue Nile

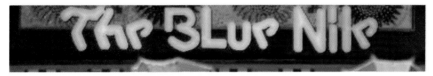

FERNDALE	ANN ARBOR
545 West 9 Mile Road	221 E Washington St
Ferndale, MI 48220	Ann Arbor, MI 48104
(248) 547-6699	(734) 998-4746
bluenileofferndale@gmail.com	bluenilerestaurant.a2@gmail.com

www.bluenilemi.com

Dining at the Blue Nile is an authentic taste of Ethiopia. Festive artwork decorates the walls, and the glow of painted lights and intricate curtains accent the ambiance with touches of the exotic. The friendly staff considers your dining experience to be their top priority, treating their customers like royalty.

The dining room features western tables and woven tables called a mesob. These beautifully decorated tables add authentic texture and color to your meal. The mesob has a woven cover that is removed when the food is ready to be served. Since utensils are not generally used (though they are available on request), a warm towel is offered to clean one's hands before and after enjoying the delicious meal.

Catering to the need for the authentic, delicate flavors of Ethiopia for larger events, including:

- Anniversaries
- Weddings
- Birthdays
- Christenings
- Church Events
- Graduations
- Reunions
- Picnics
- Holiday Parties
- Dinner Parties
- Office Parties
- Meeting

Seifu Lessanwork – Chef Bio

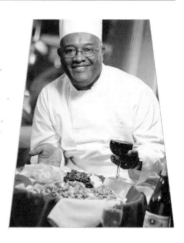

International chef & host to world dignitaries, Seifu Lessanwork brings his unique interpretation of Ethiopian traditional cuisine to the Metropolitan D.C. area. His resume spans over 4 decades & 10 countries. In 1969 Seifu joined Hilton International, where he mastered culinary & service arts in top kitchens around the globe including London, Athens, Jerusalem, Tehran, Montreal & the famous Windows on the World Restaurant in New York. In 1982, Seifu joined Chuck Muer restaurants as regional manager before establishing his signature Blue Nile Ethiopian restraint brand in 1984.

PATINO DIET Recipes from *The Blue Nile*

- **Timatim Salata** – Ethiopian Salad
- **Gomen Wot** – Collard Greens
- **Shiro Wot** – Spicy Yellow Split Peas
- **Kinche** – Cracked Wheat
- **Yekik Alicha Wot** – Yellow Split Peas
- **Doro Wot** – Spicy Chicken with Boiled Eggs
- **Yebg Kikil Wot** – Mild Lamb Stew
- **Ye Siga Wot** - Spicy Beef

Café Cortina

FARMINGTON HILLS
30715 W. Ten Mile Rd.
Farmington Hills, MI 48336
(248) 474-3033
Info@cafecortina.com
www.cafecortina.com

CAFÉ | CORTINA
SINCE 1976

Located in an Italian countryside vineyard setting in Farmington Hills, Michigan. In its nearly four decade long history, Café Cortina has consistently strived to be more than just a restaurant. Founded on the site of a former apple orchard in 1976 by the Tonon family, Café Cortina started out as a "best kept secret" restaurant that has turned into a foodie destination. Passion for people, 'true' Italian flavors, genuine hospitality, and an inspired philosophy of making a positive difference in their local community and beyond is what drives all at Cafe Cortina each and every day.

PATINO DIET Recipes from Café Cortina

- Salmone "Tireno" alle Griglia
- Pesce a Leso con Olio Erbette
- Pesce Branzino "Mediterrano"
- Vitello Tosca con Funghi al Limone
- Pesce Spada "Tireno"
- Risotto di Zucca Zafferano
- Risotto Tartufato
- Whole Wheat Fettuccine with Swiss Chard

Café Muse

ROYAL OAK

418 S. Washington Ave.
Royal Oak, Michigan
(248) 544-4749
cafemuseroyaloak.com/contact-us

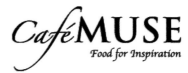

www.cafemuseroyaloak.com

David Smith and Greg Reyner opened Café Muse in Royal Oak, Michigan in March of 2006. Reyner is the creator of the unique menu, which he likes to refer to as "comfort food with a twist." A classically trained chef from the Culinary and Hospitality Institute of Chicago, his inspiration comes from the great restaurants they have visited around the world.

At the heart of the restaurant, they believe in natural cuisine. They've created a simple, European styled menu featuring as many fresh, locally produced and organic ingredients as economically possible.

They've been featured in both Esquire Magazine on The Oprah Winfrey Show. They have also been recognized the past three years as the "best brunch in Metro-Detroit" by WDIV-Channel 4 and have recently received their first Wine Spectator Award of Excellence for their unique wine list. Café Muse now features breakfast, lunch and dinner, as well as a full bar.

Greg Reyner – Chef Bio

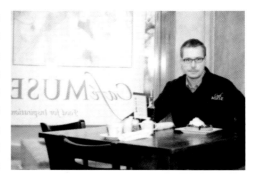

Chef Greg Reyner has always wanted to own a restaurant. Even at an early age he showed an interest in the culinary arts by spending hours in the kitchen preparing meals and honing his skills. In 1999, he chose the Cooking and Hospitality Institute of Chicago to further develop his culinary expertise. He opened his first business in 1999, a catering company called TriBeCa Catering, named after the ever-changing

NYC neighborhood.   But it wasn't until 2006 that he fulfilled his dream when he and his partner, David Smith, opened Café Muse in Royal Oak. It almost immediately became a success. Metro Times, a local Detroit publication, was the first to take notice by calling it "the best new breakfast restaurant in Metro Detroit" after only a few months of being opened.

What was his concept? Create a simple, European styled menu featuring comfort food that utilized as many fresh, locally produced and organic ingredients as economically possible. Since then, Cafe Muse has garnered recognition from both the press and customers alike. Molly Abraham from Detroit's Hour Magazine called it "one of the best neighborhood restaurants in Metro Detroit," Reyner received national attention when his grilled three cheese sandwich was named "one of the best sandwiches in America" by Esquire Magazine. This article led to an appearance on The Oprah Winfrey Show. They've also been recognized for the past three years as the "best brunch in Metro-Detroit" by WDIV, the local NBC affiliate. And after only one year from obtaining their liquor license they received their first Wine Spectator Award of Excellence for their unique wine list. Chef Reyner hopes his food - like the Muse after which the restaurant is named - will inspire his customers.

PATINO DIET Recipes from Café Muse

- Scrambled Eggs with Gruyere and Smoked Salmon
- Oatmeal Pancakes with Yogurt and Strawberries
- Spinach Salad
- Braised Lamb Shanks
- Ricotta Gnocchi with Tomatoes and Rosemary
- Tuscan Style Steak with Sauce Ammoglio

Logan: An American Restaurant

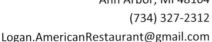

ANN ARBOR
115 West Washington Street
Ann Arbor, MI 48104
(734) 327-2312
Logan.AmericanRestaurant@gmail.com

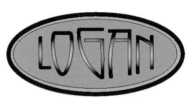

www.logan-restaurant.com

Chef Thad Gillies is chef / owner of Logan: An American Restaurant, in Ann Arbor, MI. Open since 2004, Logan is now recognized as one of the Detroit area's top dining destinations. Zagat has named it among its top ten! Chef Thad's curiosity about great food was honed during his 10 years as Executive Chef at Zingerman's Delicatessen, an icon of Ann Arbor's culinary scene. During his tenure there, Thad took a leave of absence to work in New York City. His work at Lespinasse and Union Square Café nurtured his passionate approach to French-based cooking, and it was in New York that the idea for Logan: An American Restaurant was first conceived.

Ann Arbor is a very diverse community, and Chef Thad has found a receptive public for his innovative cuisine. Increasingly, this includes scents and flavors that reflect this diversity. Drawing inspiration from Middle East/North African, Southern and Eastern Asian, and meso-American kitchens, Chef Thad develops unique spice blends, which he applies to the freshest, highest quality produce, preferably from local farmers. Then, he refines all this with classic French cooking techniques to create his unique style. Chef Thad lives in Ann Arbor with his wife, Ann Turner, and his son, Logan. Visit Logan (the restaurant!) at www.logan-restaurant.com.

PATINO DIET Recipes from Logan

- Crab and Avocado with Oven Dried Tomatoes
- Gruyere Cheese Caesar Salad
- Zucchini Carpaccio
- White Truffle Butternut Squash Soup
- Seared Tuna Sashimi
- Moroccan Roasted Chicken with a Black Olive & Butter Sauce and Oven Roasted Asparagus
- Rack of Lamb with Oven Roasted Cauliflower & Celery Root Puree

Cliff Bells

DETROIT
2030 Park Ave.,
Detroit, MI 48266
(313) 961-2543
info@cliffbells.com

www.cliffbells.com

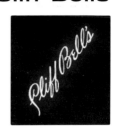

Welcome to Cliff Bell's, where a truly unique dining and entertainment experience await you. As soon as you step through our doors, you'll take a step back in time. The 1930's charm of the lavish, art-deco interior will have your friends talking for hours.

The relaxed, welcoming atmosphere sets the mood for a night not to be forgotten. Signature cocktails are ordered as the Jazz trio begins to play on stage. The quiet bustle of the club begins to come to life!

Discover this cultural gem for yourself during one of our nightly jazz sets, Sunday brunch, daily lunches, or our popular happy hour Tuesday through Friday.

"Entering Cliff Bell's is like walking onto the set of a Fred Astaire film"

- The New York Times

Matt Baldridge – Chef Bio

Flames flare on the grill, a lobster sherry reduction simmers, and steaming crocks of macaroni and cheese are pulled from the oven, all while the trumpet blasts and bass lines of jazz fill the air. This is the Cliff Bell's kitchen, home to Executive Chef Matt Baldridge.

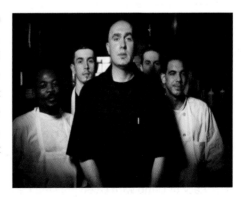

First starting his career in 1999 at The Rattlesnake Club, Matt was presented with the opportunity to help restore the kitchen of this 1930's-era club in 2008. Chef Matt has crafted a menu that combines French inspiration, soulful flavors, and the spirit of the American prohibition-era by working from menus discovered in the basement of the former speakeasy. An avid supporter of local produce and sustainable product, Chef Matt works with local growers and urban farms to develop rotating seasonal menus featuring dishes that appeal to a variety of palettes. Matt manages his staff in the kitchen, located in the lower level of Cliff Bell's, through packed-house nights of live jazz, private parties, elegant wine dinners, Sunday brunch, and one of the city's most popular happy hours.

Matt is grateful to have the opportunity to work in such a unique establishment. He looks forward to continuing his collaboration with other area chefs to establish southeast Michigan as one of the best dining destinations nationwide.

PATINO DIET Recipes from Cliff Bells

- Tofu and Avocado Timbale
- Cocoa Cinnamon and Chili Rubbed Beef Carpaccio
- Grilled Salmon with Cucumber & Daikon Radish Rolls, served with a Cucumber Basil Broth
- Seared Scallops with Oxtail Ragu

The Earle

ANN ARBOR
121 West Washington
Ann Arbor, MI 48104
(734) 994-0211
downtown@theearle.com

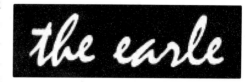

www.theearle.com

Located in an historic building in the heart of downtown Ann Arbor, Michigan, The Earle serves award-winning French and Italian country cuisine. Our wine list offers over 1,000 selections and has received the Wine Spectator Best of Award of Excellence for 20 consecutive years.

Our dining room features live jazz five nights a week. On Tuesday, Wednesday and Thursday a solo piano or solo guitar begins at 7 p.m. On Friday and Saturday our Jazz Trio plays beginning at 8 p.m.

Consistently recognized for our menu offerings, excellent service, award-winning wine list and romantic, intimate atmosphere, The Earle invites you to join us for an unforgettable evening of fine dining.

Shelley Caughey – Chef Bio

Shelley Caughey Adams is a 1983 graduate of The Culinary Institute of America and has been Chef at The Earle in Ann Arbor, Michigan since 1984. Prior to that, Shelley worked in Detroit at The London Chop House and The Money Tree. She is happily married with two children. Michael is a medical student at Wayne State University and Emily is a junior at Dartmouth College.

PATINO DIET Recipes from The Earle

- Salad de Canard – Duck Salad
- Pollo con Rosmarino e Aglio – Chicken with Rosemary and Garlic
- Gamberi al Rosmarino e Rucola – Shrimp with Rosemary and Arugula
- Coquille St. Jaques a la Crème aux Xeres – Sea Scallops in a Sherry Sauce

Red Pepper Deli

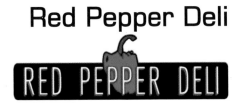

The Red Pepper Deli is an organic raw vegan eatery, striving to have the freshest food in Northville.

Eating raw is a great way to improve your health, happiness, and digestion, as well as disease preventative. Whether you go all the way or just incorporate more raw foods into your diet, you will improve in all these areas. You will be getting the nutrition and enzymes needed to live a happy and healthy life. Welcome, we hope you enjoy the food.

Carolyn Simon – Chef Bio

Carolyn Simon brought a unique organic raw deli to Northville in '08 and is dedicated to the promotion of healthy living and creating community, Carolyn has been working in restaurants for 35 years and has a great passion for food.

Having worked through her own allergies and health issues she discovered the positive impact of incorporating raw foods into her diet. She hopes the Red Pepper Deli will help others to live healthier happier lives by bringing them organic nutritious and great tasting raw food to the community.

PATINO DIET Recipes from the Red Pepper Deli

- Marinara Primavera
- Marinated Kale Salad
- Fresh Ketchup
- Emerald Isle Smoothie
- Mean and Green Meal in a Cup
- Coco Banana Smoothie

Seva

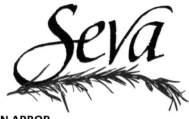

DETROIT   **ANN ARBOR**
66 E. Forest   314 E. Liberty
Detroit MI 48201   Ann Arbor MI 48104
(313) 974-6661   (734) 662-1111

www.sevarestaurant.com

Since 1973, Seva Restaurant has been serving fresh, imaginative, vegetarian cuisine in Ann Arbor, MI. The longevity of Seva is a testament to the exceptional menu which has evolved over the years and the growing interest and awareness of a lifestyle which was once considered a niche. In late 2011, a second location in the Midtown neighborhood of Detroit opened its doors. Both locations feature weekly specials, a full bar, raw juice and espresso bar.

PATINO DIET Recipes from Seva
- Farro Salad with Whipped Goat Cheese
- Peanut Kale Salad
- Guacamole
- Dr. Feelgood

Appendix

The Age of Globesity: *Entering the Perfect Storm* | Frank Patino M.D.

Glycemic Index and Glycemic Loads

TIPS AND TRICKS FOR THE LOW GI DIETER

- Avoid the following:
  - Grains and breads, with the exception of sourdough, rye, pumpernickel, and low GI specialty breads.
  - Pasta, with the exception of low GI specialty pasta.
  - Potatoes and other starches.
  - Rice, ESPECIALLY white rice.
  - Sugar and Fructose/Corn Syrup in all shapes and forms.
  - Salt.
  - Processed foods.
  - Trans fat.
  - Caffeine
  - Juice and Soda (both are quite high in sugar).
  - Alcohol, especially beer, liqueurs, aperitifs, and cordials.
- Protein should be the central focus of your meals, as meats, fish and poultry are the true "guilt-free" foods on the Patino Diet.
- Snack throughout the day on nuts, seeds, & low GI vegetables/fruit.
- Start your day with a high protein breakfast.
- Eat smaller meals throughout the day, rather than a few large meals, to keep your metabolism in "burn mode" for fat reduction.

Food	GI	Serving Size (g)	GL
CANDY/SWEETS			
Strawberry Jam	51	2 Tbs	10.1
Peanut M&M's	33	30 g (1 oz)	5.6
Dove Dark Chocolate Bar	23	37g (1 oz)	4.4
BAKED GOODS & CEREALS			
Rye bread, 100% whole	65	32g (1 slice)	8.5
Oatmeal	58	117g (1/2 cup)	6.4
Oatmeal Cookie	55	18g (1 large)	6
Popcorn	55	8g (1 cup)	2.8
Pd. cake, Sara Lee	54	30g (1 piece)	8.1
Pumpernickel bread	41	26g (1slice)	4.5
BEVERAGES			
Soy Milk	44	245g (1 cup)	4
Tomato Juice	38	243g (1 cup)	3.4
LEGUMES			
Lima Beans	31	241g (1 cup)	7.4
Lentils	29	198g (1 cup)	7
Kidney Beans	27	256g (1 cup)	7
Soy Beans	20	172g (1 cup)	1.4
Peanuts	13	146g (1 cup)	1.6
VEGETABLES			
Carrot, raw	92	15g (1 large)	1
Peas, Frozen	48	72g (1/2 cup)	3.4
Tomato	38	123g (1 med)	1.5
Broccoli, cooked	0	78g (1/2 cup)	0
Cabbage, cooked	0	75g (1/2 cup)	0
Celery, raw	0	62g (1 stalk)	0
Cauliflower	0	100g (1 cup)	0
Green Beans	0	135g (1 cup)	0
Mushrooms	0	70g (1 cup)	0
Spinach	0	30g (1 cup)	0

Food	GI	Serving Size (g)	GL
FRUIT			
Watermelon	72	152g (1 cup)	7.2
Cantaloupe	65	177g (1 cup)	7.8
Papaya	60	140g (1 cup)	6.6
Kiwi, w/ skin	58	76g (1 fruit)	5.2
Orange	48	140g (1 fruit)	7.2
Grapes	43	92g (1 cup)	6.5
Strawberries	40	152g (1 cup)	3.6
Apples, w/ skin	39	138g (1 med)	6.2
Pears	33	166g (1 med)	6.9
Peach	28	98g (1 med)	2.2
Grapefruit	25	123g (1/2 fruit)	2.8
Plum	24	66g (1 fruit)	1.7
Sweet Cherries, raw	22	117g (1 cup)	3.7
NUTS			
Cashews	22		
Almonds	0		
Hazelnuts	0		
Macademia	0		
Pecans	0		
Walnuts	0		
DAIRY			
Ice Cream (Lower Fat)	47	76g (1/2 cup)	9.4
Pudding	44	100g (1/2 cup)	8.4
Milk, Whole	40	244g (1 cup)	4.4
Ice Cream	38	72g (1/2 cup)	6
Yogurt, Plain	36	245g (1 cup)	6.1

Food	GI	Serving Size (g)	GL
MEAT/PROTEIN			
Beef	0		
Chicken	0		
Eggs	0		
Fish	0		
Lamb	0		
Pork	0		
Veal	0		
Deer-Venison	0		
Elk	0		
Buffalo	0		
Rabbit	0		
Duck	0		
Ostrich	0		
Shellfish	0		
Lobster	0		
Turkey	0		
Ham	0		

Take a look at Mendosa's list of low carb variations for variants of bread, pasta, and other food types that are GI/GL friendly:

http://www.mendosa.com/low_carb_low_gi_foods.htm